MAY I BE HAPPY

MAY I BE HPPY

A Memoir of Love, Yoga,
and Changing My Mind

CYNDI LEE

DUTTON

DUTTON
Published by the Penguin Group
Penguin Group (USA) Inc., 375 Hudson Street, New York, New York 10014, USA;
Penguin Group (Canada), 90 Eglinton Avenue East, Suite 700, Toronto, Ontario
M4P 2Y3, Canada (a division of Pearson Penguin Canada Inc.); Penguin Books Ltd,
80 Strand, London WC2R 0RL, England; Penguin Ireland, 25 St Stephen's Green,
Dublin 2, Ireland (a division of Penguin Books Ltd); Penguin Group (Australia),
707 Collins Street, Melbourne, Victoria 3008, Australia (a division of Pearson
Australia Group Pty Ltd); Penguin Books India Pvt Ltd, 11 Community Centre,
Panchsheel Park, New Delhi–110 017, India; Penguin Group (NZ), 67 Apollo Drive,
Rosedale, Auckland 0632, New Zealand (a division of Pearson New Zealand Ltd);
Penguin Books (South Africa), Rosebank Office Park, 181 Jan Smuts Avenue,
Parktown North 2193, South Africa; Penguin China, B7 Jiaming Center, 27 East
Third Ring Road North, Chaoyang District, Beijing 100020, China

Penguin Books Ltd, Registered Offices: 80 Strand, London WC2R 0RL, England

Published by Dutton, a member of Penguin Group (USA) Inc.

First printing, January 2013
10 9 8 7 6 5 4 3 2 1

Copyright © 2013 by Cyndi Lee

 REGISTERED TRADEMARK—MARCA REGISTRADA

LIBRARY OF CONGRESS CATALOGING-IN-PUBLICATION DATA

Lee, Cyndi.
  May I be happy : a memoir of love; yoga, and changing my mind / Cyndi Lee.
    p. cm.
  ISBN 978-0-525-95384-5
  1. Hatha yoga.   I. Title.
  RA781.7.L44 2013
  613.7'046—dc23
                                        2012021472

Printed in the United States of America
Set in Weiss Std
Designed by Jamie Putorti

For Mary and Dzolly
and
my beautiful Millie

Arising

Vinyasa has three parts: arising, abiding, and dissolving. And the dissolving of one thing is the arising of the next. Every day turns into night turns into day. Winter becomes spring becomes summer becomes autumn becomes winter. Waves roll in and slip back out; tides ebb and flow. Every breath is like this. Every life is like this.

Each flower buds, ripens, and blooms, wilts and fades away. The leaves fall to the earth and create the ground for a new plant to grow.

The Sanskrit word *vinyasa* means "to place in a special way." It means that everything is connected and the sequence of things matters. It means that every action, thought, or word that arises now is planting the seed for future fruit. "In a special way" means the unfolding of life is logical. If you plant a tomato seed, you will get a tomato. If you plant an apple seed and you wait long enough, you will get an apple tree. And if you plant a hard thought, you will get a hard heart.

———•◆•———

"There's something wrong with my knees." This thought bubbles up like a lava lamp blob pinched off from the rest of my consciousness, which is still oozing around the depths of my jet lag nap. Deep murky sleep is normal for me after I cross the international date line; but having a sideways furrow across my knees is not normal, and it hurts. My Buddhist studies have taught me that thoughts lead to action and as my mind registers this thought about pain, my body responds naturally. I reach a hand out of my fetal position to rub the tender spot and fall asleep again.

I wake up with my hand still on my knee and look around the room. The furniture makes me think of England. Lolling over onto my back, I stretch my legs straight up to the ceiling. This might not be normal for other people but most mornings you can find me somewhere in the world with my feet up in the air. I'm a yoga teacher and turning upside down is part of the gig. I slowly circle my ankles, which tend to swell on long international hauls and then, just to get a little abdominal work in, I stretch my arms up to the ceiling. Taking hold of the gathered elastic around my ankles, I pull my sweatpants down to my thighs to check out my lumpy knees. With one hand still on my ankles, my other hand reaches over to the British-y bedside table and grabs my red cat's-eye glasses to take a closer look.

Aha. With my two upside-down legs now aligned side by side, I see a horizontal indentation tracking across both knee caps. I'm only five-foot-four-and-a-half inches tall but these Western-sized legs were too long for the leg room provided by a coach ticket on Cathay Pacific. Fifteen hours of having my knees smushed against the metal dowel lining the seat-back pocket had evidently changed the topography of my knees. Remembering how my flattened breasts always spring back into shape after a mammogram gave me hope that my crushed knee flesh would similarly re-plump, returning to normal soon. Recovering normal is part of the gig, too, when you are a traveling yoga teacher.

People think being a yoga teacher means you are always chill and never grumpy; your mental outlook is radical contentment and your body is outrageously flexible in a sexy way. But that is not the case; not for this yoga teacher anyway. Well, actually, I am extremely flexible. That part is true. But the other parts come and go, depending on how much sleep I get, what I eat for breakfast, how much money I have in the bank, what's happening between me and my husband, David, or how many time zones I crossed in the last twenty-four hours. Perhaps that sounds quite ordinary and distinctly non-yogic, but without all that normal stuff in my life, I wouldn't be a very good yoga teacher. How can I help others grow and transform if I haven't done it myself?

Another thing that many people don't realize is that yoga teachers are not born as yoga teachers. We are not born standing on our hands or doing the splits—although I did all those things in my backyard when I was a kid and then just never stopped. Many American yoga teachers, like me, are regular people who have had the great fortune to be introduced to the path of yoga in our lifetime.

For me, doing yoga is pure fun. I love twisting and bending, inverting and jumping on my yoga mat. I thrive on the hard work of standing on one leg while keeping my face soft and open. I find bending over and folding in half a delicious release. I especially enjoy the ending of each class when the teacher instructs us to lie down and rest, telling us this is the most important part of the practice. The clean, sweaty feeling I get from yoga is physically global, purifying me inside and out. Every part of my body is opened up and then put back together, reintegrated into a better shape than before yoga. From the first day of practicing, I could feel my inner organs getting toned along with my triceps and quadriceps. My heart got stronger, my stamina improved and one day I discovered that it had gotten easy to lift heavy objects over my head, such as a carry-on bag into the overhead bin of an airplane.

Most surprising is that I began to focus on the immediate experiences I was having in yoga at the same time that I was having them, a bigger view of the practice rather than just being satisfied with short-term goals, such as being able to touch my toes or turn upside down and inside out. I had been studying ballet since I was seven, so I was very familiar with extreme movement scenarios. What was different about yoga is that it isn't really about the external activity; it's about what's going on inside. It's not about what we do as much as how we do what we do. I began to understand that this is the part of yoga that really matters.

I studied yoga with as many masters as I could get to, including the great yoga master B. K. S. Iyengar, who told me and the other 899 yoga students in class that day, "I've spent almost my whole life observing what happens to my sternum when I press my big toe down." In other words, yoga is about more than moving the body; it is a template for understanding that every thought really does become speech, which turns into action. If the yogi practices with this awareness, she will also become curious and conscious about the results of her actions, making her a better wife, mother, friend, and businesswoman.

Hearing my yoga teachers talk about this eventually led me to the path of Buddhist meditation, where I learned and practiced specific skills for negotiating all the different mind states that arise on any given day. That doesn't mean I am always successful. It means I am working on it, in just the same way I am still working on becoming more adept at doing the yoga postures. I want my mind to be as flexible as my body, and my heart to be as open as my hip joints. And once you get flexible and strong, you can't stop the work. You have to keep practicing with more refinement, more awareness, more skill in order to maintain and grow your abilities and your understanding. I know all this and have made it my long-term goal—which in yoga means lifetimes—but like anyone else, I sometimes feel defeated by circumstances.

These days there is a lot of pressure on yoga teachers. We can't just lead people through a sequence of asanas. We are expected to always act positive, be smart, and to look, if not glamorous, at least extra-good. For one thing, people take pictures of me all the time, usually when I am bending over to adjust a student's yoga position and my butt is looming large; or when I am exhausted and wearing my funkiest yoga clothes dragged from the bottom of the drawer; or when I am giving a precise verbal instruction that makes my brow furrow into a stern, unappealing expression. And then, of course, these candid cell phone photos are posted on someone's Facebook page for all the world to share. Okay, okay, that was a little rant about the pressure I feel, but please don't get me wrong! I love my gig and almost everything about it.

For the last eighteen years I've been a full-time yoga teacher and I'm grateful for the various opportunities that have come my way, such as being invited by the popular American Buddhist nun Pema Chödrön to lead "yoga breaks" for the nine hundred meditators attending her inspiring teachings or being hired by MTV to stand up in front of a New York hotel ballroom full of rowdy, hung-over sales reps and transform their heckling into five minutes of quiet meditation—and have them actually like it!

One time I even gave a one-on-one yoga class to Prince Andrew, who, like me, happens to be extremely flexible. He was staying with one of my private clients at her posh Sutton Place apartment in Manhattan. At first, I wasn't sure if it was okay to touch him since he is royalty, but then I just decided that it was fine because, in that moment, I was his teacher and he was my student. It was my job to adjust his posture, so I placed my hands on his ribs and helped him deepen his twist. He was very polite and thanked me for that adjustment, which I thought was pretty nice and normal for a prince. Perhaps the monarchial decorum can be more relaxed when he is on this side of the pond.

My home base is New York City, where I teach yoga at OM yoga Center, the studio I founded in 1998. I'm convinced it was a combination of right time–right place and my particular style of rigorous, intelligent, and fun yoga classes that made my studio an immediate success. Within a few years my teaching career outside the studio also began to rise. In 2007, I was still beginning my international teaching career, but in that year alone, I taught yoga on four continents and in six countries, twelve U.S. states, and fourteen U.S. cities—and I visited my mom in Dallas five times. My recognition was growing and my jet lag was starting to add up.

I slid off the bed and managed to scuff my way over to the window with minimal knee bending. I rubbed my eyes and ran my fingers through my hair, which felt fat and curly, bloated just like my ankles. Even in the air-conditioned hotel room I could feel a bad hair day coming on, and then I remembered why. I was in Hong Kong.

My student Margie had warned me that Hong Kong in June was crazy humid; she stressed the word *disgusting*. A native of the place, she'd recommended staying inside at all times. But from my high window perched over the harbor I was charmed by the wooden sampans with colored sails, the kind of boats I'd only seen in black-and-white films. I wanted to get out and see magical old Hong Kong. My hotel was cushy but it wasn't the real world; it was full of ultra-sophisticated Chinese men and women dressed in Western clothes who looked like they never had a bad hair day.

Should've listened to Margie. The pungent smells from street cook pots and the sticky, sweet temple incense glommed together into a noxious potion that you could almost see hanging static in the thick, polluted air. I felt sick to my stomach instantly. The 90 percent humidity caused the straps of my sandals to rub my feet raw after walking only half a block. It had been a mistake to wear new sandals anyway, but I wanted to look good for my big adventure in Asia. I'd also gotten my hair freshly cut and colored and picked up a few new summer dresses, like the one that was sticking to my sweaty thighs right now.

After dragging myself up and down crumbly stairways that seemed more decrepit than charming, I finally plopped down on a curb, between lines of hanging chickens and hanging laundry. I slipped off my sandals and put my head in my hands. As a yoga teacher, I'm an expert in breathing techniques. I wondered if it was possible to draw in slow, deep breaths without actually inhaling any of the stinky, wet air. I tried it while David went down an alley, in search of a taxi to take us back to the sanitized refuge of our hotel.

Surprisingly, the South China News reported that the air quality that week was the best it had been in quite a while. I had come to Hong Kong to be a featured presenter at the very first international yoga conference in Asia. Although there were at least thirty-five other faculty on the program, being invited to this inaugural event was significant. It meant that my work was considered valuable enough to be included in the new mix of yoga that was spreading across Asia.

No longer the exclusive domain of Indian gurus, the packed conference schedule offered five days of flowing yoga, static yoga, fusion yoga, couples yoga, power yoga, slow yoga, quiet yoga, and hot yoga. Special lectures would be given on anatomy, breathing, chakras, and meditation, as well as workshops for injury prevention or therapeutics for those who already have injuries. Yoga students could clean their innards with a day-long detox program or conquer their fears by turning upside down.

At the faculty welcome dinner the night before, I was greeted by a sari-clad woman who touched my third eye, leaving a sacred smudge on the spot between my eyebrows. Ushered past a row of red lotus candles, I stepped out onto the terrace just in time for the Hindu puja, a fire offering and supplication to the gods for an auspicious conference. Woozy from jet lag, I plopped down on a silk cushion in the back row and tried to relax without falling asleep to the gentle droning of the monks' chanting. Following a period of silence at the end of the prayers, our conference host stood up and extended an upward palm toward the apartment's dining room. "Please, everyone, help yourself to dinner." Ready to escape the heat, I peeled my sweaty self off the terrace floor, walking through swirls of incense smoke on my way back indoors.

Once inside I started to perk up from the stun-gun air-conditioning and realized I probably needed to eat something. After hitting the buffet, I took my plate of Indian food over to a couch and sat down to schmooze with some of my yoga teacher buddies. For several of us, this was our third yoga conference teaching gig in as many months and we started making jokes that we were a yoga teacher touring band. Hugs, kisses, and a bit of harmless patting ourselves on the back: "Fancy meeting you here." "Didn't we just do this last month?" Yes, we did and I realized that attending a party in a far-off land with monks and yogis was becoming a very normal thing for me.

There were also lots of presenters I hadn't met before from Australia, Thailand, Indonesia. It was cool to see the different ways that people presented themselves, wearing anything from luxurious silk saris to tight jeans and Ganesh T-shirts, or monks' saffron robes. There were noses pierced with tiny diamonds and ankles tattooed with coiled serpents representing the potential for awakened energy. One woman was heavily draped in layers of white robes, and I thought she must be sweating under all that fabric. Adjusting the straps of my new summer dress, I shook hands with esteemed scholars of Sanskrit, Vedanta, and Tibetan Buddhism.

Finally our local colleagues rang a gong and officially welcomed us, telling us they were honored by our presence in Hong

Kong and joking that the air was especially good that week because of all the clean, fresh energy we visiting yogis had brought to town.

It was slightly intimidating to be part of such an all-star yoga-teacher lineup and naturally I hoped to make a good impression. I knew I'd been invited because of my reputation for bringing wisdom and humor into my smart, soulful, and sweaty yoga classes. But my popularity gave me no confidence. On the outside I was friendly and positive but inside I felt bad, grumpy, and agitated; distinctly not yogi fresh. It wasn't just the challenging climate. The problem was more about the weather in my head; a storm was going on in there. I was obsessing on my body and what people might think about it.

It was those damn mirrors everywhere—in restaurants and subways, along the hallway of our hotel, on all three sides of our bathroom. Every time I turned around, I saw my face, my hair, my belly looking back at me and I didn't like what I saw.

Riding the mirrored elevator back up to the room after our visit to old Hong Kong the day before, I was surrounded by my reflection, showing me that my body was just not good enough. Frizzy hair was the tip of the iceberg. My appearance clearly did not measure up to the yoginis on the cover of *Yoga Journal.* "Maybe those models are airbrushed," I thought, trying unsuccessfully to give myself a pep talk.

Arriving at our floor, I grabbed my upset stomach and dashed to the bathroom. As I washed my hands I saw my mirror image again, front, sides, and back. That meant I could see my butt, which somehow seemed massive. I could see my arms,

which looked squishy even though I'd been doing extra workouts with my trainer!

Yogis don't necessarily need to do other forms of exercise,
but for me joining the local gym was an opportunity to work
out in an anonymous setting, something I longed for those days.
With the recent death of my father I had gained weight, which
I knew was part of the grieving process, but I also knew it was
time to move through it. To do that, I felt like I needed to be in
a space other than my studio, a place where no one knew me
and I could be tired and look tired and feel flabby and not care.
The very first day I went to the gym I was offered a free personal training session with Smith. The thing is, I knew Smith.
So much for anonymity. He had been an OM yoga student for
years but it actually worked out well, because he didn't really
want to talk to me either. He didn't want to get to know me or
become buddies. He just wanted to get me into great shape.

Smith took me on as a serious project, offering to give me
personal training sessions in exchange for free yoga classes. Four
days a week he made me curl my biceps, dip my triceps, run for
miles on the treadmill, and cycle standing up. He even had me
slithering around on my elbows and dragging my belly like a
lizard, an exercise I'm pretty sure he invented but which was
highly effective for engaging the triceps and abs. His workouts
made me sore for days, which I considered positive, having been
brainwashed from an early age to appreciate what my ballet
teacher called "profitable pain."

Having a trainer was good for me in other ways, too. I teach
so many people all day every day that having someone else tell

me what to do and then making sure I was doing it right was nourishing for me. I was a willing and obedient trainee, completely open to whatever Smith suggested, especially since I thought it was working. But now I wasn't so sure.

Ever ready to feed my self-critical nature, I went for a closer-up inspection in the magnifying mirror, where I discovered an unwanted line of grayness marching through my honey-colored dye job. The final insult! My roots were already showing and I'd just gone to the salon right before this trip! Arggh!

I was frustrated and mad—mad at my body for not keeping up its part of the bargain, especially since I had done everything I could:

✦ Hair dyed—check

✦ Nails done—check

✦ Facial—check

✦ No dairy/gluten—check

✦ Gym workouts—check

✦ Yoga—check, check, check!

So, why didn't I look better? Why couldn't I look exactly the way I wanted to look, even for a little while?

Seeing my eyes in the mirror, I was almost shocked by the guilt, shame, and failure they reflected. Whoa. This intense state of mind was freaking me out.

As I walked back into the bedroom, David felt my vibe and asked, "What's the matter with you?"

"I feel so fat! I'm wrinkled and I hate my hair." I spit out the words. "I can't stand to look at myself."

"So . . . that's why you have been so mean to me lately," David replied. "You are being mean to yourself, too."

Too bad I didn't know then what I know now. I didn't know that international travel bloats you. I didn't know that jet lag makes for fuzzy thinking and sleep deprivation kicks up your cortisol, creating waist fatness. I didn't know that if you just relax and drink a lot of water, things will be different in a couple of days; it's all impermanent.

I didn't know that none of this matters anyway. I didn't know that trying to keep myself looking good—hair dyed, body firm, wrinkles smoothed—wasn't going to make me any happier. It wouldn't make people like me better or enhance my career in any meaningful way. It wouldn't make me more attractive to my husband or bring me a drop of joy. I didn't have a clue that worrying so much about all that stuff was actually my own personal form of self-torture; that focusing on it so much only made me feel worse, not better. I didn't know that taking care of myself wasn't the same as actually caring about myself. I didn't recognize that my lifestyle tactics were just my habitual way of experiencing what my Buddhist teacher calls suffering.

Turns out that David, like all good husbands, was a better mirror than the ones on the wall, reflecting back both my outer actions and my mental state in a way that finally woke me up. Ugh. I saw this whole scenario as something way too familiar.

For my whole life, too much of my sense of self-worth has been wrapped up in how I feel about my body, a body that has never seemed quite good enough. The other day a guy friend of mine said, "You have such nice, juicy hips. Why do you hide them under tunics and baggy sweaters?" At first I waffled, defensively telling him how much I love the feeling of loose clothing and the boxy, draped silhouettes of Asian fashion. "Sure, sure," he said, "but I still want to know why you're hiding your beautiful bottom." Pressed, I finally blurted out, "Because since the first day I can remember I've been told that big behinds must never be seen. And even though that makes me mad and sad and I don't believe it and I applaud every woman who doesn't go along with that baloney, I still . . ." And then I ran out of steam. It felt familiar to get spun up about this topic and then have nowhere to go, because, as usual, I wasn't walking the talk. I hate admitting it but I don't have the courage to be the first big butt on my block to not care what anybody thinks of me.

Ever since Gloria Steinem came to my high school in the seventies I've known this attitude sucked. Queen Anne High School towered above Seattle, perched atop the highest hill in the city. One of the many brick buildings constructed after the Seattle fire of 1889, it was so old that the steps of the up-and-down stairways were permanently indented from decades of student's saddle shoes. This ivy-covered landmark building was built in the Classical Revival style, which I suppose was intended to tell everybody from the top of Queen Anne Hill all the way down Skid Road to Elliot Bay that Seattle boasts excellence in classical public education. You could see the school for miles in all directions. Perhaps less a matter of pride was that fact that you could also see the students every night on the local five o'clock news. The opening credits showed protesting QA high school kids burning the American flag outside the lunchroom, while the news show's opening music played the urgent sound of a Morse code tapper. Up until 1967, the classical education was standard fare but things shifted when Mr. Hall became the principal.

I went to Queen Anne High for sophomore, junior, and senior years and those three years happened to coincide with most of Mr. Hall's brief tenure. He was a little too radical for the parents but that was one of the main reasons we liked him. We also liked that he banished study hall. He changed it to "free period," which I interpreted as meaning you were free to do whatever you wanted. By the time I was a senior I had manipulated my schedule to be totally free of anything resembling science or math, but I did like to go to journalism class in the morning, where I hung out with Tina. She was the front page editor of the school newspaper and I was the back page editor and together we drove our journalism teacher crazy. He complained that we were too giddy and giggly. Of course, that just made us laugh more. After journalism, I had my first free period followed by lunch followed by another free period, which added up to about three hours of doing whatever I wanted. Tina and I would usually get in my car and drive to the University district for pizza and then go to the bead store to make daisy-bead hippie bracelets.

Our first year of high school was 1968 and we were still heavily influenced by our parents: hers were strict Catholic and mine were liberal Protestant. Contrary to our journalism teacher's impression of us, Tina and I were actually thinking girls, and in those days, there was a lot to think about for young high school women.

That didn't mean we weren't both excited and flattered to be asked to model for the high school fashion show. Sharing a dressing room at Jay Jacobs, a cool Seattle store that provided the clothes, we took turns trying on skirts and tops and alter-nately complimenting each other and criticizing ourselves. I slipped a daisy-print shift over my head and posed in front of the mirror.

"That is adorable! You look so cute in that dress!" raved Tina. I also thought I looked cute in that dress but I didn't say so. That would simply not be acceptable.

Instead I would say something like: "Really? You think this looks okay on me?" And then she would say something like: "Yes, you should definitely model that dress."

This kind of conversation went back and forth between us, me telling her what she looked good in and her telling me what I looked good in, and we had started to pile up the outfits we wanted to model for the show when we began to notice a lot of noise from outside. The dressing room was on the second floor with a little window that looked across the main downtown plaza toward the monorail. Pulling the curtain aside, we looked out and saw a huge, roiling crowd of people on the sidewalk below. The intense energy was exciting and scary at the same time.

"It's an antiwar march," said Tina.

"Oh yeah, I think my dad is down there somewhere."

"Your dad is in a protest march?"

"Yes!" I was proud of my dad and even bragged about how,

as a minister, he willingly wrote conscientious objector letters for any boy who asked him.

Tina was equally shocked when I told her that not only had my dad marched with Martin Luther King, Jr., but so had my mom! This was the same year that reproductive rights for women were recognized as a basic human right. Her Catholicism and my Protestantism clashed hard on this.

"Go home and ask your mom if she would get an abortion if she found out she was pregnant," Tina dared me.

So I did and my mom told me that, yes, she would get an abortion.

Okay, maybe she didn't exactly say that. I'd like to ask her about that now but she is too far gone into dementia. Even if I had asked her a few years ago when she could still remember a thing or two, I imagine she would have said, "Oh, Cyndi" in the same way she did when I was in college and I told her that I had done LSD. That particular "Oh, Cyndi" meant she didn't believe me. She thought I was just trying to shock her, which I was, even though what I said was true.

So I must include the possibility that this memory is not 100 percent accurate. Maybe what happened is that when I asked her if she would get an abortion she said something like, "Oh God, I don't want another kid!" But whatever she actually said, the message I heard was clear—nobody else can or should tell you what you can or can't do with your own body.

My mom expressed that opinion often—even though she also criticized her younger, hipper coworker for never wearing a bra. And I believe Mr. Hall wanted his students to contemplate these kinds of contemporary conversations because he used his new concept of free period to bring in controversial speakers, providing a powerful, worldly education for his students. When I was sixteen and seventeen these speakers affected me deeply. I spent one week boycotting Safeway after hearing César Chávez speak about migrant workers, and when Gloria Steinem came to our school, my life was changed forever. Here again, my memory might not be 100 percent reliable. I think it was Gloria. I know for sure there was a remarkable and important woman who came to our school's free period, and this is what I remember.

She was beautiful and smart and clear speaking. She talked about how the traditional role of women was expanding and inspired us to take advantage of any opportunity. She told us that no choice was wrong except the one that was imposed on us. She said whatever choices we made in the future—stay at home, go to college, get married and have babies, or become career women—were all valid paths for us as young women. I didn't know exactly what I wanted to do but I knew that I did not yet want to be a housewife and a mother. I didn't want to step around toys and tricycles, like I did when I was babysitting. I wanted to get out of the house. I wanted to see the world. I wanted to dress in pretty and sharp outfits and go to work with people who respected me and made me feel smart and valuable, just like my mom did when she went to the office every day. I had big ideas and a creative drive and a sense of undirected ambition. I was seventeen and I believed I could do anything I wanted. Since then I have done most of what I've wanted, but doing whatever you want and feeling however you want are not the same thing.

Somehow I got stuck in a place where being respected and

liked for what I could do was important but still not enough. I never felt 100 percent satisfied with any positive feedback if it didn't include how I looked, yet being complimented on my looks wasn't enough either. I didn't want to be just a pretty face but I wanted to be noticed for my pretty face. I didn't want to be sought after for my body but I was envious of other women's bodies that I thought were better than mine. And since jealousy is a bottomless pit, there was always a better body invading my comfort zone. Eventually I learned to control my body through dance, yoga, and politics, but I hadn't understood that what needed to be controlled was really my mind.

Gloria Steinem knew that the main change we needed was an attitude adjustment, a re-positioning of women within our culture. That's why she became a Playboy Bunny. Criticized for being too pretty—as if that meant she couldn't be taken seriously as a force for women's rights—she turned those comments upside down by getting a job where her uniform was a leotard with a puffy tail and ears on her head. By exposing the sexism of that gig she showed that women can take ownership of their own beauty, sexuality, and brains.

Of course, there's a reason why she is Gloria Steinem; it has to do with vision, bravery, and a willingness to tirelessly spread the message that no one's body—women, men, children, or animals—is an appropriate political war zone.

Forty years later, I understand this. I love this. I love Gloria. But back then, I was caught in a riptide that flowed in two opposing directions. One wave was moving forward, taking me and my friends and even my mom toward becoming more confident beings in the world. I set my sights on living a life that mattered to me and felt respect for all women, including those who had a different vision for their future. I was smart and I expected to be treated as an intelligent and worthwhile person, even if I was planning to have a career as a dancer and, hopefully, make a living from how I moved my body through space. And, sure, I wanted a bra when I was twelve, but by the time I went to college, that thing was long gone and I never got another one until I was fifty-five and noticed that my breasts were finally starting to droop. At which point I thought, why not? The imprints from Gloria were still there—I didn't care if you could see my nipples through my sweaters. But I didn't want anyone to think that meant something that it didn't. I was free but I wasn't cheap.

And then there it was, that other tide, the backward-moving undertow that sliced through my self-esteem and told me that what other people think about me matters. My personal perception problem was so typical that it became a completely normal part of life. My girlfriends and I talk about what is not quite right about our bodies, how we can't wear this or that because we just don't have the right legs or waist, or because it makes us look fat even when we aren't fat. We are all way too good at denigrating ourselves with each other, just like Tina and I did in that Jay Jacobs dressing room when we were fifteen-year-old smart goddesses with tremendous potential to be anything we wanted. Our only obstacle was that we could only really feel good about our appearance—and in turn, ourselves—when it was confirmed by others.

This was no small thing because the seeds that were planted in my mind at that age have grown up into a full-blown adult body grudge. Most all of my friends know this syndrome well and consider it a normal thing for our self-esteem to be based on how we *feel* about how our body *looks*. Not on our actual embodied experience, which might be strong or grounded or capable, but how we feel about our physical self—the size and shape of our breasts, the firmness or not of our abs, our dress size, and how much we weigh compared with each other.

Even a woman like me, who has been always been physically active—tree-climber, cheerleader, modern dancer, aerobics instructor, yoga teacher—has spent a lifetime chipping away at my own self-confidence by comparing my body to a fictionalized PR ideal based on celebrities and fashion photos. But even though I know those images are unreal, the imprints are too deep to be easily swept away.

Why do I care so much about such shallow concerns? It's not as if this is all I have to do or think about all day. I have serious interests, my own business to run, a committed spiritual practice, and thousands of students who look to me for guidance and inspiration. What they don't know is that in the background there is always a grumbling, rumbling, complaining voice in my head that tells me that my body needs work.

———— • ◆ • ————

As a little girl, I never really thought about my body. I was my body and my body was me. I didn't have any brothers or sisters but I was always able to keep myself company because I had a good, strong body that took me on lots of adventures. A typical day found me scaling the apple tree in our backyard, flying down hills on my skateboard, or standing on my dad's feet as he waltzed me around the living room. Heights and speed attracted me and even though I dislocated my elbows, skinned my knees, and even cracked my head open one time, nothing ever slowed me down. I was born to move.

When I was seven, I was secretly in love with Bill Sutton, who was a drum major for the high school band. Our families were friends, and Bill thought it was fun to have me as his little groupie. When I heard the band practicing in the school field across from our house, I was so excited that I raced across the street without looking and was hit by a car. I ended up with fifty-six deep stitches in my right calf and strict instructions from the doctor not to do anything active for the rest of the summer. That didn't last long.

Stuck in my room, I turned my bed into a trampoline, which not only stretched my sutures, leaving me forever with a wide silver scar, but also broke the bed frame. My mother had yelled at me to stop bouncing on the bed a million times. But at this point she was grateful I was still alive. Over and over she recited, "That car could have killed you," followed by a lot of dramatic sighing. She already knew it was a lost cause; I was never going to stay still.

More injuries were in my future: wiping out on a hairpin turn while wearing cut-off jeans on a high school ski trip landed me in the emergency room with a deep gash in my knee. One sexy college night in the southern California canyons, I busted a couple of toes when I tripped literally while tripping on acid. Ballet lessons and modern dance performances led to ankle sprains, sciatica, torn spinal ligaments, whiplash, and lumpy purple bruises in every place imaginable. If I got bumps along the way it was no big deal—I was nothing if not resilient.

My fourth-grade pals decided one day that I shouldn't exercise so much. They thought I was too skinny. They made me eat seconds on our favorite school lunch of chili and cinnamon rolls and refused to let me play kickball. Instead, two at a time, they took turns holding each other's wrists to create a palanquin for me, insisting I ride everywhere to avoid burning up even one calorie.

In truth, I wasn't really too skinny and I certainly wasn't fat. I was just a very alive little kid with bright energy and a sense of adventure. I wanted to see what was around the next corner or on the highest branch. I wanted to ride the wind and hang upside down, and I had total confidence that my body could always take me wherever I wanted to go.

If I close my eyes and sit quietly now, I can remember how it felt to be me then. My body was my best friend. We had so much fun together every day and just as with my other friends, it wasn't about looks but about feelings. I don't remember ever feeling too big or too small. I felt good. I felt right. I felt free and joyful and full of movement. I didn't know then that it could ever be different.

———— •◆• ————

My yoga students are sitting on blankets with their legs bent in an extra-challenging version of a crossed-leg position. Their right ankles are balanced on their left knees and their left ankles are placed directly below their right knees, in a pose called Agnistambhasana, or Stacking Fire Logs. A few people like this position, but for the most part, they look at me like they just sucked a lemon. Time for me to give them a big-picture view.

I ask, "Have you ever disliked someone that you didn't even know? Maybe a person at your office that you've seen from a distance and, for no reason at all, you just don't like them?"

People nod, a sheepish admittance that they've all been there.

"And then, did it ever happen that circumstances put you together and you ended up really liking each other a lot? Maybe even becoming great friends?"

A few eyebrows go up and heads nod as they get the message: Stacking Fire Logs might not be your friend right now, but maybe if you relax your idea about it, that could change.

I talk about this all the time when I'm teaching yoga. Since every body is different it just makes sense that some people can naturally do certain poses, while other ones seem completely impossible. You might be desperately struggling to lift your leg an inch off the floor while the perfectly ordinary person on the next yoga mat has somehow managed to toss a knee over his shoulder without any drama at all. I want to encourage people not to solidify what they think they know about themselves and any one pose; to instead rethink their relationship with the ones they've already labeled as enemies.

Many of the students are regulars at my New York studio, OM yoga Center. They've heard me talk about this before. Maybe the reason they are smiling at me is that they recognize this is a lesson I'm trying to teach myself.

———— ✦ ————

By sixth grade, my body innocence had started to shift along with my hormones. I got some new ideas from 16 magazine, and Donna Reed's wispy daughter, and especially from my friend

CeeCee Carlott and her big sister. The main message was that if I wanted to fit in, I had to pay vigilant attention to my appearance.

I did my best to get the right look, but somehow I was always out of sync. At eleven, I still had a girl's un-curvy body although I was dying to be like voluptuous Barbie. Then, just when my teenage body started rounding, the "in" look was all about flat-chested Twiggy, with her boy hips and boy hair. I could never quite hit the target, but I was already a slave to the junior high message—no matter how my body looked, there was always room for improvement.

Boobs were a good place to start. CeeCee and I had been trying to get our boobs to grow ever since we found a *True Confessions* magazine stuffed under the couch cushions at Gil Larkey's house. We knew for a fact that it belonged to Gil's grandmother, who was our number one audience—in fact, our only audience. A sensuous, slouchy kind of lady with bedroom hair, her suggestive vibe was a total turn-on to us pre-sexualized tweens. Stuff that our moms would not want us to be doing just cracked her up, like semi-risque dances involving bumps and grinds and flow-y scarves, or dramatized versions of the illicit love stories from *True Confessions* that might include kissing each other on the lips. The back of the magazine had a cheesy ad for a bust enhancer, some kind of gadget that you hold between your hands and squeeze. We really wanted to send away for one but, of course, we didn't have any money. We also didn't have any breasts to enhance but by the time we were in junior high, we understood the principle of how the thing worked. Who needed the gadget? We figured out that we could join our hands in prayer and push, push, push in a rhythm that engaged our chest muscles. Results were inconclusive, which meant it was worth it to keep trying.

By 1968, we were in high school and the tide that undercut our natural little-girl-body joy was in full force. No longer were we having fun exploring our bodies and movement and feelings. Now we were clearly focused on the goal: We wanted our chests to get bigger and the rest of us to get smaller. Before school we drank Instant Breakfast instead of eating something and after school, we sprawled across our parents' living room floors running rolling pins up and down our thighs just in case the rumor was true and that really did make your legs get thinner.

As the daughter of the minister of a big downtown church in Seattle, I had the added pressure of upholding the purity quotient of my entire generation. There were comments from some of the older church members when I started rolling up my waistbands in seventh grade—a popular method for shortening your skirt. Fortunately my mom was a pretty cool minister's wife, telling the church biddies, "A short skirt is not a crime!"

Millie's fierceness did not tolerate anyone criticizing me, her only child. I might step out of the good-girl box in little, insignificant ways, but that only made her more proud of me for being a kid with chutzpah. In the meantime, she counted on me being reliably afraid of the things she and my father had brainwashed me against, such as older boys and motorcycles. As soon as she was able to convince my dad that I was old enough to stay home by myself, my mom went back to work as an executive secretary.

Each morning, before getting in the car to go to work, she

stood on tiptoes, the back of her feet lifting out of her high heels, to hide the house key on top of the garage door ledge. Each afternoon, when I got home from school, I stood on the tiptoes of my saddle shoes. Just able to touch the edge of the key, I would flip it off the ledge and catch it as it fell down, to let myself into the house. My mom never suspected that her good-girl daughter brought her boyfriend home with her most days. My basement bedroom was next to the garage so it was easy to hear the car coming down the driveway. Over the three years of high school Mick and I got pretty fast at disentangling our limbs, smoothing our clothes, and composing ourselves before she stepped into the house. Because my mom thought I wouldn't want to do anything that a non–good girl would do, she just assumed that I wasn't doing anything with my boyfriend that she would not approve of. And on Fridays she was right.

That was payday. My mom's contribution to the family money scenario was buying the groceries for each week. I would help out by going to the store with her and then loading up the backseat with paper bags full of Rice-A-Roni, Pop-Tarts, iceberg lettuce, and Neapolitan ice cream. Then she would turn to me and say, "Well, I still have a little bit of my paycheck left and you know what? This money is burning a hole in my pocket!"

She would drive us out to the Northgate Mall, famous for being the first retail shopping mall in America (and less famous for being the mall parking lot where my dad taught me to drive). We'd make a beeline for the fabric store, where we walked side by side down the middle aisle. Rows of fabric on our right and left, we each ran a hand along the top of the end bolts. Walking slowly, if we felt something we liked, we would stop and unroll it, running it through our hands with as much relish as if it were food. Textiles nourished us. If we liked the color, we might buy it. If we liked the texture, we might buy it. If we liked the texture and the color, we definitely bought it. We didn't have to know what we would make out of it. We just bought fabric the way other people might buy shoes.

We loved having new clothes that nobody else had. In fact, that was our policy. The feel for fabric was in my mom's fingers. She intuitively understood how it folded together and ended up in three-dimensional shapes and she could do this with or without a pattern, even on short notice. When I got an unexpected invitation to a girls' club party, my mom and I agreed I absolutely needed a new dress. We dug into our fabric stash and pulled out a couple of yards of blue-and-green madras plaid and half a yard of plain turquoise cotton. Exactly one hour later, my mom put on the finishing touches with the iron-on hemming tape—only to be used in this kind of fashion emergency—and I slipped on a groovy new tent dress that no one else would be wearing at that party.

Millie and I had new outfits almost every Sunday, including mom-and-daughter dresses, with an après-church matching sports shirt for Daddy. I was always proud of the clothes she made for me, except for one time when I was about twelve.

When Mom made me a Carnaby Street–style shift with bust darts and paraded me around church, I thought I would die. Right at the front of the sanctuary she said, "Show Mrs. McHargue the new dress I made you!" I slowly spun in a circle wishing I could corkscrew right down into the floor, sure that everyone was staring at my non-breasts. As far as I was concerned, my mom might as well have screamed to the whole congregation, "Look at little Cyndi's chest!"

Even though I had been squeezing my pecs since a year earlier, when they actually started to bud, it seemed so embarrassing. I didn't know if I wanted them or not. But what I did want was a bra. My poor friend Carol had just been given her first training bra as a Christmas gift and we all talked about how embarrassing it was for her to open it up in front of the whole family, including her big brother! That was horrible, but at least she ended up with a bra, which definitely increased her coolness quotient among our little crowd.

I also wanted pantyhose and kitten heels and ruffled collars. I liked being a girly girl just as much as I liked climbing trees, but I just didn't understand curves. And already I was resentful that anyone would notice me for my body or judge me by my looks. I didn't know that was called objectification and I didn't know how to recognize mixed messages. I just knew that getting attention for how I looked was the way to be accepted, and at the same time, wanting that kind of attention was not an acceptable way for a good girl to be.

In eighth grade my friends threw me a surprise party, and my mom redeemed herself by buying me a new pair of jeans, taking them to her sewing room, and tapering them to a perfect fit. Like today, skintight jeans were essential if you wanted to be cool. This was long before the invention of jeggings and stretch denim, so everyone spent hours sewing up side seams to make their jeans super tight. We even left a little opening at the bottom of the seam to solve the problem of how to get your feet through your pants. But I had another problem with my jeans. My hips were bigger than my waist. Jeans that might fit my waist would never have fit my thighs and vice versa. Without my mom's waist tucks, my pants would be the right size at the hips but the waistband fabric would have stuck out like a hula-hoop.

Clearly I must be a freak if pants fit me like that. I had no idea that boys' jeans—which was the only style that was made back then—don't taper in at the waist. I became obsessed with the part of me that went out because it seemed so big. And everybody knew big is not what you want your body to be, right?

Little did I know that one of the hottest icons of that era had exactly the same problem. Thirty years later, I found myself standing on a round pedestal in the Armani dressing room on Fifth Avenue. It was shortly before my second wedding and I'd lost about twenty pounds, which was good except that my waist was still considerably smaller than my hips.

Kneeling at my feet with pins in her mouth, the in-house tailor told me, "Don't feel bad that your hips are bigger than your waist. That's why I have a full-time job here. Everybody has this problem. Even Sophia Loren! I have to take in her clothes all the time. She is always telling Armani, 'Dahling, I refuse to wear your clothes any longer unless you make them fit a real woman's body.'"

In high school, I finally began to understand that some curves were good, but unfortunately, those weren't the ones I had. I'd learned that guys like breasts but also that they didn't think mine were big enough. Neither did my drama teacher, who suggested falsies for the bodice of my *Hello Dolly!* costume. At the same time, my dance teacher was not so subtly encouraging me to diet, since, "You know, my dear, the stage adds ten pounds." I was five foot four, barely weighed one hundred eight pounds and size small was baggy on me. Yet evidently I was too big in some spots and too small in others—talk about a lose-lose situation. The relationship with my body was just not much fun anymore. A source of wrongness in so many ways, my body was no longer my friend.

———— ✦ ————

Looking back to the time of Sophia's heyday, I wonder why I never had the opposite thought—that my waist was extra tiny and my hips were average. But it never occurred to me to think that. Along with my girlfriends, I'd already developed a typical American female's critical assessment of her own body, and it always came up lacking. To me, *curves* was just another word for "fat."

That thinking was still with me in 1984. It was Larry Kirwan's birthday and we were all at St. Marks Bar on Eighth Street and First Avenue to help him celebrate. Larry Kirwan and Pierce Turner had a band called the Major Thinkers, which was Cyndi Lauper's opening act on her Ready-in-Five-Minutes tour. I danced for both bands and Pierce wrote the music for my dance company, called XXY Dance/Music. We were all starving dancers and musicians with no money ever but loads of ideas and energy and joy.

When I think back on that time it seems like we were always either in that bar or Blanche's on Avenue A or the Holiday on St. Marks between First and Second, and I wonder how I ever managed to do all that dancing, but I seem to recall that hangovers were part of the creative process.

Just say that we were pretty comfortable hanging out in bars and when one of us girls came up with the idea of taking her clothes off as a birthday present for Larry, we instantly decided that we would all do it!

We huddled together in the ladies' one-seat, one-sink bathroom with walls painted black and started undressing. We bumped butts as we reached down to pull off our pants and knocked elbows turning around to unzip each other's dresses and the whole thing had us in hysterics. And then, one by one, we got qualms. Even though we were all in our late twenties with gorgeous dancer bodies, we each had one area that we didn't want to expose. We certainly were not prudish. But about half of us wanted to hide her boobs and the other half wanted to hide her butt. The girls with bigger breasts wanted to keep their bras on because even though big boobs are always popular, my chestier friends were all critical of their breasts—too floppy, too low, you get the picture.

That surprised me since I'd spent my entire adolescence and early adulthood wishing I had bigger breasts and secretly hoping they could still grow in my twenties. I tried not to hate my friends with big boobs but I was definitely jealous of them and part of me was glad they didn't like their breasts. Did I subconsciously feel that if they didn't like their bodies it somehow made my body better? Or it made my own negative body image acceptable?

That night I didn't mind showing my small, perky breasts but no way was I going to go out there bare-assed, even though my underpants were practically nothing. It seemed like we were all more comfortable with exposing the part that we thought was small and firm. Anything round or squishy must remain under cover.

We paraded back out to the bar in our bras and high heels, panties and Doc Martens, high on the outrageousness of it all and a little bit turned on, too. I'm sure on some level we knew we were wielding a kind of power, feminine sexual energy power, but mostly I think we related to our bodies in terms of what size or shape seemed to be in style. Rather than a source of power that I could be proud of and take ownership of, exposing my body was more like giving something away—Happy birthday, Larry!

I guess we took too long in the bathroom, though, because when we arrived at Larry's bar stool, he was gone. He was barfing around the corner on St. Marks Place and missed the entire display, which made the whole thing kind of fall flat. We got plenty of unwanted attention from the other patrons, though, and we scurried back into the bathroom to cover up. It occurs to me that on some level we really did know what we were doing. The magical power spots of our bodies, the seats (no pun intended) of our female energy were what we had to give but even then, half drunk, half stoned, and half delirious with youth and East Village craziness, we knew that we weren't willing to give it all up. I'd done practically everything else in a bar—snorted coke, danced on the bar, sung at the top of my lungs, fondled, been fondled, and gotten famous for being an excellent mooner, so why not just take it all off? But the inhibitions had limits.

Maybe we knew we were hot, but we didn't know we were magic. We didn't know that our natural beauty and sensuality were more valuable than the size or firmness of any particular square inch of flesh. I'd like to think that we were making some kind of conscious statement, but really it was just a spontaneous expression of that uncontained time in my life—full of raw, organic, sexual, youthful, highly stimulated life energy. But as fun as it all was, there were still feelings of inadequacy, jealousy, and negative self-esteem hiding under the covers of every hot night with a guy in the band.

When I told this story to my old friend Mary, she told me that these days she is jealous of her own ex-body. I laughed, sort of. Honestly, I think she and I both feel a little bit sad that we weren't more proud of our beautiful young bodies—bodies that we would kill to have today.

The thing is, I didn't even know I had a bad attitude toward my body. It wasn't that obvious, in large part because it was the same attitude that all my girlfriends had about their bodies. Nothing had changed from the days when Tina and I had been high school models. Not one of us would ever say right out loud "I look good in this outfit" or "I love the shape of my body." Your friends might tell you that you looked good, but of course, since everyone said that to each other, it wasn't a reliable compliment.

It was simply the accepted way for women to talk about them-selves with each other. All of this behavior was so normal that it took many years for me to realize the harm I was doing to myself. It was pernicious, and yet so subtle, that it didn't make me stop eating or become anorexic or bulimic or addicted to exercise. I just felt like an un-cool person with a wrong-shaped body who wasn't crazy about mirrors.

———— ✦ ————

Touring as a backup dancer with Cyndi Lauper required serious creativity in the area of body, hair, and clothes. We girls really did just want to have fun, and to prove it we wore tomato-red bangs or hot-pink hair swirls to match our combat boots and layers of petticoats. The show was called the Ready-in-Five-Minutes Tour because we were always late. One reason is that Cyndi and I liked shopping.

"Hey, Cyndi."

"Yeah, Cyndi?"

She showed me a handful of ruffles. "I can't wear this, but I think it would be cute on you."

I don't know how she found this vintage place in the coun-try outside of Philly. There were piles of old clothes every-where, the kind we liked, with lots of ruffles and plaid and white petticoats, old-fashioned bathing suits and boy shorts. Heaven! Our policy was to never wear only one skirt at a time. A good look was at least three skirts over a pair of pedal pushers or boy shorts, with a camisole on top and only one very long earring.

I piled so many taffeta skirts on top of multiple crinolines that I felt like a Michelin man. Even though I thought I was fat, I was so skinny that almost everything vintage was too big for me, but if there was something there that would fit me, Cyndi would find it.

"Here—try this skirt on over that bathing suit. Adorable!"

Cyndi Lauper was an expert at unearthing cute, kooky items and generous in sharing what she thought looked good on me. We had a few hours between arriving at the venue and when we had to be back for the sound check, which we thought was plenty of time. But back at the arena, it took a while to get all those layers on just right and if the show started late because we had to put on more eyeliner or change the shoelaces in our Doc Martens, that just made the audience even more eager. The manager had to deal with the union guys but since he was also the manager for Lou Albano of World Wide Wrestling fame, we didn't worry about it too much.

Basically, I didn't worry about much anyway, except, of course, my hair and my body. My favorite haircut was Little Lord Fauntleroy on one side and almost shaved on the other. Running down the middle fell one long strand that went all the way to my upper lip. Believe it or not, it was a pretty sexy look on me.

In fact the whole experience of being on tour was sexy, especially the hot affair I had with the bass player. He was very into his look—always wearing sunglasses onstage and minimal shirts that showed off his hyper-muscular arms and chest. I wasn't the only person who got to see his naked chest, but I was one of the few who got to see his naked eyes after the gig. He also had a high-maintenance rock 'n' roll hairdo. He was very willing to spend an entire day sitting in a chair to get those long black braids down to his waist.

But most guys I know aren't like that. I know some of my men friends don't always agree with me, but it seems to me they are not obsessed with their bodies in quite the same way that we women are. By the third date, I knew I was crazy for David but I was pretty shy to show it. And since I'd only been separated from my first husband for a week, I was very out of dating shape and didn't really remember how things went in that department. Near the end of the date, when I couldn't help myself anymore, I bravely reached out and touched his hand. He seemed to like that. As I gently stroked the hairs on his big fingers, I asked him if he had a hairy back.

"A hairy back?!"

"Yeah."

"I don't know."

"You don't know? How can you not know if you have a hairy back?"

"Who knows that? I mean, how can I tell if my back is hairy? It's behind me and I can't see it."

That was so cute. I was really falling in love with him. I didn't care if he was hairy or not, and honestly, I could hardly wait to find out for myself how hairy his back was or wasn't.

So I said, "Well, don't you ever stand backward in front of your full-length mirror and then swivel your head around so you can see your back and check out your butt?"

"No."

"Oh."

Most guys I know are all like that. They might have a beach ball for a stomach, firm and very round, or a blubby spare tire situation. But they just don't get too worked up about it. And body size, shape, and furriness is rarely an obstacle to lovemaking with the lights on. To them, sex is like a trendy nightclub—a-see-and-be-seen event. Although mostly guys want to see you and it's only us women who don't want to be seen.

My friend Jeffrey told me that his girlfriend constantly berated her body and eventually it just wore him down. He asked her, "If you really have such a horrible body, what does that say about me, your boyfriend? If I like your body—but you hate your body—what do you really think about me? Do you even like me?" The whole drama upset and confused him, when he just wanted to feel loving and close to his girlfriend, who he thought was beautiful.

One day my husband grabbed me as I stepped out of the shower. He ran his hands up and down my body, clearly liking what he was seeing. He said, "When are you going to write an article called 'I Hate My Body but My Husband Loves It and Wants Me to Let Him Play with It'?"

Another wakeup call from my husband-as-mirror. This I-always-think-I'm-fat thing may be a women's issue but it's our husbands—and everyone around us—who get the fallout. My husband looks at me and sees a beautiful, luscious woman but then he looks in my eyes and sees a person who is dissatisfied, judgmental, and not that much fun to be with.

I think Jeffrey's question is valid for all of us. If we don't love ourselves, can we love our husbands? Are we telling them we are unlovable? Does this attitude create a loop of un-lovability?

———— • ◆ • ————

Most of my yoga classes begin with some kind of breathing exercise. I might invite the students to equalize their inhalation and exhalation to balance active and receptive tendencies. Some days we practice sharp exhalations and passive inhalations as a kind of purifying breath. The most basic, and yet most advanced, breath work is simply cultivating breath awareness, which naturally brings one's mind into one's body, creating a harmonious sense of presence and grounding. Pretty much everybody feels better after a few minutes of doing that, even if they didn't feel bad before.

"On your next exhale, unfold into your first Downward Dog of the day. Stay steady here for a few breaths. Take a moment to experience what your breathing is like, right now, in this upside-down position. Can you take interest in the sensation of the breath? Not the concept of the breath, but the actual texture of each inhalation? The warp and weft of each exhalation?"

I let a few moments pass as I walk among the students, moving between the rows of mats. I'm not touching anybody yet. It's too early for that. If I'm asking them to check in with their experience as it is, without manipulating anything, I don't want a hands-on adjustment from me to imply that anything about them should be different right now.

Today I'm offering a specific exploration, one that I've been drawn to a lot lately and I hope the students aren't getting bored with it. I didn't know that someday soon I would meet Louise Hay, a wise woman in San Diego, who would tell me: "We only attract people to us that we can help." I just had to trust that since they kept showing up for class, they must have been getting something they need from this experience.

Along with touching and not-touching, part of skillful yoga teaching is working with the rhythm of silence and non-silence; I start talking again.

"I'm sure I'm not the only woman here who steps on the scale every morning to figure out how I should feel about myself that day."

Mark, a longtime student of mine, pops his Downward Dog head up and gives me a dirty look.

"Okay, I get it. Why am I leaving out the guys? I know you do that, too."

He affirms this with a grunt. I continue.

"The thing is, we are using the scale as if it were a mirror. We allow that little box to tell us how we should feel about ourselves today. If we like the number it shows us, we feel good and if we don't like the number, we have a little dark drama moment.

"Of course, this wouldn't be a problem if we didn't believe that the information we receive from external feedback is fixed and real. But we do, so we meet that by allowing our response to be equally solidified. We see a precise number on our digital scale and we accept it. 'That's how much I weigh and now I feel this way. Period.' We look in the mirror and based on what it reflects, we accept that this dress does not look good on me. Period.

"But, have you ever weighed yourself before you went to bed and then again as soon as you woke up in the morning? Isn't it funny that you lose weight overnight, even though you've just been lying in bed for hours—and then you gain weight again during the day? We're made of water so, of course, any kind of accurate feedback loop is going to need to be more fluid."

Okay, I've ranted long enough. Their arms are getting tired and they are ready to move. A good yoga teacher knows what to do by looking at the students. My living, breathing dots of awareness are starting to fidget, so I tell them to move into plank pose and exhale their knees, chest, and chin to the floor. Inhale into baby cobra, exhale child's pose, inhale, and round up into Vajrasana, Basic Goodness Pose.

"Does this resonate with anybody or am I the only one who has this mirror-scale issue?" They crack up. We're all on the same page.

"The good news is that we're here. Yoga offers us a different mirror—the reflective surface of the breath. Come back into Downward Dog and sensitively walk your feet to your hands. Slowly round up to standing, feeling every single vertebra as if you were doing a walking meditation all the way to the top of your spine."

The students stand at yogic attention—calm, centered, bright, open—waiting for the next instruction. I can tell that for that moment, no one is feeling fat or thin or wrong in any way. They are not unsatisfied and neither am I. For the moment, we are in the middle of our experience, no need to lead or follow.

———— ✦ ————

People often ask me if I fell in love with yoga as soon as I took my first class. I was eighteen and it was 1971 in southern California, so naturally my hippie college offered yoga classes at the traditional crack-of-dawn time slot. It's more likely that I fell in love with the yoga and art teachers who took us on a retreat to the Joshua Tree desert and taught us about purification and Indian art. It was a fun time to be young; the birth control pill was easy to get, and HIV/AIDS was unknown. I was crazy in love with my life as a full-blown vegetarian-cooking, TM-meditating, hitchhiking-to-Berkeley, *Siddhartha*-reading, hash-smoking, orgy-making hippie. Since I frequently partied half the night anyway, I thought it was kind of relaxing to take a yoga class before going back to the dorm for some sleep.

Clearly, I wasn't as serious about yoga as I was about dancing. Eight years later I tightened the ribbons on my toe shoes one last time and graduated with honors from one of the most respected university dance departments in the world. I tucked my MFA under my arm and moved to New York City as the token performance artist recipient of a fellowship to the Whitney Museum of American Art. I ditched my dance shoes and pink tights for bare feet and sweatpants, taking contact improv classes from influential movers such as Simone Forti and Danny Lepkoff. Studio rental was about three dollars an hour, but since the Whitney gig paid only sixty bucks a week, I started teaching yoga to support my dance habit.

For next to nothing I shared an apartment with another dancer on Avenue B and Fifth Street in the East Village, and I soon became a fixture in the downtown modern-dance world. Eventually I was invited to perform my own choreography in theaters around the world, which brought my work to the eyes of video producers. My first commercial gig was choreographing the music video of Cyndi Lauper's "Girls Just Want to Have Fun" for which I was paid one hundred twenty-five dollars. It was 1983. My hair was blue, and I still taught yoga on the side.

In 1984 Cyndi Lauper's video won the first-ever award for Best Female Video at the MTV Video Music Awards and that brought me more work. Over the next few years, along with my choreography partner, Mary Ellen Strom, I choreographed music videos for many artists, including Rick James, Simple Minds, and Apollonia. We did spots for *Sesame Street's* Children's Television Workshop and choreographed the videos for the *Dirty Dancing* soundtrack. We were super excited to perform live with Cyndi Lauper on NBC's short-lived Friday night version of *Saturday Night Live*, especially since the show was hosted by Steve Martin. One crazy night, while we were in San Juan choreographing some videos for Latin pop star Chayanne, we even threw together a dance segment in about fifteen minutes and performed it live on the popular Puerto Rican TV show *Sabado Grande*. This was all a lot of work and great fun, but not much money or, really, much of anything meaningful to me. I considered myself a serious dancer, dedicated to making art, but after a while that felt empty, too.

My last dance concert was at the famous Saint Mark's Church in-the-Bowery on Second Avenue and Tenth Street, which is also home to the Poetry Project, Danspace Project, and Incubator Arts. Founded in the midsixties, Saint Mark's was host to artists such as Philip Glass, Allen Ginsberg, Yoko Ono, Anne Waldman, John Giorno, and Sam Shepard. It was Philip Glass who first introduced me to his guru, Gelek Rimpoche, and by the early nineties I had a new love, the Buddhadharma. Yoga and dance had flip-flopped for me and I was now completely passionate about my yoga practice with the result that all my dancers were adept yogis.

The concert at Saint Mark's was called *The Beat Suite*. It opened with a dancer in Parsva Bakasana, Side Crow Pose, which means that she was basically curled up sideways into a ball, one hip balanced on her arms with her feet hovering off the floor. If that wasn't challenging enough, she stayed like that for five minutes, now and then slowly coming down out of the pose and shifting to the other side. It was an expression of the stability and strength that I was beginning to experience from my meditation practice.

The highlight of *The Beat Suite* evening was a group of short dances choreographed to songs written by Allen Ginsberg, known as the poet laureate of the Beat Generation. Allen was also a student of Gelek Rimpoche and a longtime resident of the East Village. We ran into each other on the street all the time and he'd always give me a big sloppy kiss that practically left my whole face wet. As my dharma brother and fellow downtown artist, he was happy to let me use his music for my concerts, sometimes even showing up in person to sing his songs and play his harmonium while we danced.

The concert opened with *Dunderhead Hoover,* a solo I performed while telling a Buddhist fable I found particularly inspiring. The story goes that a not-very-bright young man (aka a "dunderhead") had a yearning to become enlightened. He had been enrolled in his uncle's monastery but, unfortunately, he was not smart enough to grasp the teachings and in the end was kicked out of the school. Then his luck changed because the Buddha himself just happened to be walking by and saw the poor fellow crying by the side of the road. He brought the young man to another monastery and gave him the job of sweeping the temple floor. A simple job, for sure, but Buddha added one particular element. As he moved the broom back and forth, the dunderhead was told to recite these words, "Sweep the dust and sweep the dirt. Sweep the dust and sweep the dirt."

In the teaching of the story, dust represents the concept of attachment, and dirt refers to aversion. The moral is that if we can sweep away our desire to hold on too tight to what we like as well as our urge to push away things that we don't like, we will find ourselves in a place of equanimity, awake and clear.

The happy ending of the story is that the dunderhead became enlightened through repeating these positive phrases, along with right motivation and true commitment. It shows we have the potential to become enlightened, too, because we all have Buddha Nature or Basic Goodness at our core. Our practice is not a magic pill to bring us to enlightenment, but a process of creating the causes and conditions for that awakening to happen if we do the work.

Each time I repeated these phrases to the audience at Saint Mark's, I swung my body across the stage, rolling and bounding up, again and again, stage right to stage left to stage right, hoping to embody the notion that conscious repetition can result in creating new imprints. This is the basic notion of all practice— whether it is yoga, meditation, or sweeping the floor—and the path that can lead us from negative habits toward positive patterns of thinking and behaving. I liked that idea a lot but didn't know myself well enough to see the negative ruts that I had already created and was constantly solidifying with my repetitive self-judgment.

This was my professional dancing swan song because, for one thing, it wasn't fun to perform anymore. My old love of movement was overshadowed by needing good reviews and making sure that influential people from the art world were in the audience so that the necessary fund-raising work could continue. But it was more than that. My mind had turned to the dharma. I wanted to practice meditation every day. I wanted to teach yoga full-time. I was starting to be as interested in what was going on in my mind as I was with my body. I was already stepping onto the path even though I didn't know where it would take me or how hard it would be.

———— •◆• ————

Wake-up calls like the one I got looking at my gray roots in the Hong Kong bathroom mirror can be destabilizing. Right away my mind started racing—could I get a quickie dye job in the hotel; how long would it take; how much would they charge? These thoughts spun around and around, a mind tornado of criticism, and soon enough, everything else felt wrong, too. When my husband asked, "What's bothering you?" it was like a ray of sun piercing a cloud. He cut through the thunderstorm in my head, and for a moment anyway, my hard heart melted. I really didn't want to be cranky to my husband just because I needed a dye job. How ridiculous!

I didn't have a solution but I was starting to know I had a problem. Where do you go with that? Perhaps it is ironic that I was in the land of Buddha, on a breezy ferry ride back from Lantau Island, home to a ten-story-tall Buddha sitting in lotus and smiling gently to remind me of the blissful peace that comes from within. But instead of feeling peaceful, I was suffering.

Even at the time, it felt arrogant and whiny to glorify my feelings by calling them suffering, when there are so many less fortunate people in the world. But in his first public teaching at the Deer Park, the Buddha himself said that everybody, everywhere suffers. When I first heard Gelek Rimpoche speak about the Buddha's view of suffering, I was in my mid-thirties and didn't relate to that teaching at all. Even though I had a short temper, a frustrating dance career, a week-to-week-paycheck life, and an alcoholic (now ex-) husband, I really didn't think I was suffering. And, of course, I was right. In the grand scheme of things I was affluent, healthy, surrounded by friends, options, and lots of laughs. Suffering, I thought, is what happens in India and Africa or maybe Appalachia.

But as my studies in Buddhism deepened, I learned that the "suffering" the Buddha was talking about might more accurately be translated as dis-comfort, dis-ease, a constant background of dis-satisfaction. "If only this one thing were different, I could be happy, free, find love, relax" is one version. Or alternately, "If only I could be happy, free, find love, relax, then this one thing would be different"—which is just the opposite side of the same coin.

With permission from Gelek Rimpoche, I'd begun integrating Buddhist kinds of ideas into my yoga classes. My unique approach to yoga is an organic blend of all my practices and interests, which include dance and Buddhist meditation. After teaching full-time for a few years this work clarified into a method I began to call OM yoga and which was the basis for my book, *Yoga Body, Buddha Mind.* The Buddhist teachings of wakefulness, compassion, impermanence, appreciation for this precious life, and the importance of making friends with yourself—these were the lessons I brought into my yoga classes at OM yoga Center.

So, instead of asking when the beauty salon at the Hong Kong hotel opened, I started asking myself different, deeper questions: Why I am so freaked out by these little gray hairs? I have never been one to hide my age, even now that I'm over fifty. So what was the problem? Why should I feel bad about myself for being myself? Is my happiness so delicate that its very existence depends on the color of my hair? Do I really care what other people think about me? Or what I think other people think about me?

Asking myself these questions is a form of svadhyaya, or self-inquiry. I tried to contemplate these issues without engaging in any story line, but honestly this whole hair-dyeing thing was making me feel claustrophobic. I remembered one of the definitions of suffering, or dukha: sitting alone in a dark, cold room. That's just what I felt like—isolated and stuck, in a place with no way out.

Every time I thought about my gray roots I was reminded of a hair-coloring tip I'd learned from one of my yoga students after she stood on her head in my sixth-floor walk-up apartment on St. Marks Place. Even though she was the VP of a major record label, she liked slumming it down to my little place for the refuge of a private yoga class. We worked on her inversions against my closet door. After ten deep breaths, she came down out of the pose and rested in Balasana, Child's Pose. As I gave her a grounding hands-on adjustment I noticed a dark smudge on the mat.

"Ooh, there's a little schmutz on your mat, Nina."

She sat up and laughed, rubbing her fingers along the part in her hair. "That's my secret for when my roots start to show. I cover them up with mascara until I can get a hair appointment."

Very clever, I thought, but when that memory came back to me, I knew I didn't want to go there. It's not that I had a problem with coloring my hair. Turquoise, jet black, lemon yellow, and a bold sunset of fire engine red, orange, and gold melting into sienna—this is only a partial list of colors I've dyed my hair over the last thirty years. Surprisingly, it hasn't been a big topic of conversation, but that's because I've lived my entire adult life in New York's East Village, a neighborhood where artistic expression includes all body parts. Even after I hung up my leotard and became a professional yoga teacher, I still had a peacock-tail color wheel hiding under my ponytail.

I don't know when my goals shifted but eventually coloring my hair was no longer about looking different but about looking the same. All my friends colored their hair, except for one who defiantly let her gray hairs go wild. Ugh. Those witchy strands were coarse and crinkly and I thought she looked messy.

But the mascara trick depressed me. I intuitively realized that the answer to my problem was not to do something more. It wasn't going to be about fixing anything or adding on, even if it was only a little brown mascara. The accumulation approach to life is like trying to overcome obstacles by dressing them up instead of meeting them head-on. Ironically, it is also the best way to perpetuate a problem.

Maybe that was another thing I'd learned from meditation, which is a reductive activity. It's a practice of letting go and doing less; an undoing rather than a doing. Just as we can consciously practice developing the qualities we want to become, we can also consciously let go of whatever it is we don't want to be anymore. And what I didn't want to be anymore was a fake brunette with blonde highlights who spends hundreds of dollars and hours to maintain the facade. I was going to the salon every three weeks and it wasn't working anyway. When I thought about having to dye my hair forever just to keep the nagging voice away, I felt trapped. Maybe that was a tipping point.

What if I tried something radical, a completely opposite approach—what if I actually let my hair go gray altogether? I'd first considered the idea a few years back and brought the idea up to my hairstylist. Her response: "Well, you know, you will look a lot older . . ." That was disappointing, but I wasn't surprised. After all, why would she encourage her clients to stop using her coloring services? I decided I needed to ask around a bit more.

So I told my husband I was thinking about it. He liked the parts about saving money and about me feeling more authentic. Being a guy, he said, "Let's do some research." So he and I started a game called GA: Gray Alert. Whenever we saw a woman with totally gray hair we whispered, "GA" and then gave a thumbs-up or thumbs-down. We saw lots of older hippie women who had the same hairdo they'd had since 1971 (thumbs-down) and we saw elegant women with stylish cuts (thumbs-up) and we saw cute, gray-haired Barbies with ponytails and bangs (me up, him down). My research showed that the messy, witchy look is a result of scraggly hairdos, no matter what age or color.

And I also discovered something else important. There aren't a lot of role models for women my age to be inspired to look our age, to feel our age, to even act our age! Helen Mirren, Kathleen Sebelius, Emmylou Harris, Donna Brazile, Jamie Lee Curtis are a few, but there aren't many others.

And what about aging in yoga? Isn't that supposed to be one of the realms where seniors are venerated and the wisdom of the elders is appreciated? So where are those gray-haired yoga teachers in *Yoga Journal?* Well, there are some but they are in their eighties and nineties and Indian and male.

When I was studying dance and on the way to my professional dance career, I was in love with Isadora Duncan, who didn't ever care what anyone thought of her and lived by the motto "Truth Is Beauty." She was my role model in every way, including wearing toga-like clothing and Greek sandals. I aspired to be free of cultural restraints like Isadora, but I just couldn't ever do it. In the end, Isadora was alone and sad and broke, which was not how I want to end up.

Yet the message of our society seems to be False Is Beauty and I don't want to go there either. When my movement interest merged with my spiritual quest, I fell in love with yoga. Fortunately, this is also an area with inspiring, brilliant female role models, but now that I thought about it, did any of them have gray hair?

Then one day during this contemplating-going-gray phase I found myself in a van that was taking me to the Denver airport, after I'd finished my teaching at the *Yoga Journal* conference in Estes Park, Colorado. I looked up at the seat opposite me and there she was!—my new role model, Angela Farmer. Exquisitely beautiful, she has long, wavy silver hair that is magical and completely natural. We introduced ourselves and after a little small talk, I screwed up my courage and said, "I love your hair. I'm going to stop dyeing my hair and let it go gray, too." Her husband, Victor, right away said, "Oh, you must! It will be gorgeous!"

That pretty much clinched it for me, and I decided to go for it. It was a big letting-go of what I thought I needed to do to be happy, of a habit that had become a burden, of a way of thinking about myself. I reminded myself that's what yoga is about—letting go of whatever prevents us from being our most authentic self—and it helped me stay committed to my decision.

I made a plan: stop coloring my hair in November, and then two months later, go to India. I was already signed up for a "Footsteps of the Buddha" pilgrimage through Nepal and northern India. Could there be a more perfect time to stop obsessing on one's hair color or body? By the time I got back to New York I'd have a couple inches of gray. Then I would get a super short haircut and take the first step toward doing less and being more real. Just thinking about it made me feel better, it really did.

I didn't tell anybody about my hair project but I just stopped getting it dyed and went to India. And you know what? Nobody noticed the gray roots coming out anyway.

———— • ◆ • ————

"Congratulations to everyone for figuring out to come to yoga. It's such a brilliant system for aligning our skin, muscles, and bones and leading to radiant health!" I love saying this so much that my arms fly out like I just stuck the landing off an Olympic balance beam.

"So, what do we call it when we do this thing we call yoga?"

"Practice."

"Yep, and that really is what we're doing—we're practicing for later; for the other parts of our life when we're not 'doing' yoga. Everything we do creates imprints, so when we practice yoga we have the opportunity to consciously choose what we are imprinting.

"Everyone, please close your eyes and take a moment to think about what you want to cultivate."

Many students already have their eyes closed but I can tell they've been listening. With this little assignment in mind, they all sit up a bit straighter, place their palms down on their knees and gather their minds.

I love looking at them. There are so many different kinds of people in the class—seventy-two-year-old Nanette, wearing bracelets up to her elbows, is on the mat next to twenty-two-year-old Nate, a long-haired martial artist who looks like Jesus. There are short, tall, thin, and zaftig bodies of all ages and colors and nationalities. Trying to be invisible over in the corner is the movie star who just got married to Daniel Craig, although right now she doesn't look anything like a Bond girl. Which is another brilliant thing about yoga class. It is a great leveler. No one is in a business suit or hard hat, even though I happen to know there are many top-level executives here and that guy in a black leotard and tights who looks like a retired Merce Cunningham dancer is actually a construction-site foreman. Right now everyone is just sitting on the floor in some relaxed variation of sweatpants and T-shirts. The honesty and vulnerability of each person touches me deeply.

Even though most of the students had to zoom to get here on time, negotiating the subways and schlepping through the highly populated neighborhood of Union Square, by now they are relaxed and open to what I'm saying. They know that the little talks I give at the beginning of class help them let go of the stress of their day and drop into an earthy sense of composure.

"So, what is it that you want to practice?"

They are very willing to participate.

"Being present."

"Mindfulness and compassion."

"Not pushing myself."

"Being with the breath."

I feel a teacherly sense of satisfaction about their thoughtful answers.

"And, have you noticed that everything shows up in your body—agitation, contentment, hunger, joy, lust, restlessness, boredom—and that's just in the first Downward Dog, right?"

The students get little Mona Lisa smiles on their faces when I say this because, of course, we've all experienced this.

"Turns out that the body is the perfect vehicle for getting to know yourself better, which means that these poses give us lots of chances to practice whatever we want. We can shift away from uncomfortable feelings such as agitation and boredom by noticing the feelings arise and then do what they always do—pass. When we engage in that process we are also developing mindfulness and compassion at the very same time.

"Let's try it. Come on up into the first Downward Dog of the day and then just stay there."

I had to say that last part really fast before the students started wiggling around in their Down Dog Poses. It is a common habit among all yogis to tinker with positions, especially at the beginning of class. It can feel good to move hips side to side or tread the feet in place to get the kinks out. But I'm giving a different lesson right now, one that is about making friends with whatever arises—which really means making friends with yourself.

"Even if you are dying to adjust the position of your hands and feet or anything else, stay still for just a few breaths."

I caught some of them just in time. I can feel that they are itching to move, but at the same time, people are willing to try something new. They've developed a confidence in what I have to teach them.

"We all have a tendency to want to fix things but right here, right now you have a chance to take a naked look at your situation without managing it or changing it in any way.

"Notice the adjustment that you want to make and notice if that is the same one you always make when you first come into Downward Dog. And notice if you really need that adjustment or if it is just a habit."

As I look at the sea of Downward Dogs, strong legs and arms diagonally reaching away from each other, creating a V-shape with their bodies, I can feel a settling spread through the room.

Because I want to model the notion of friendliness through my teaching, now I tell them, "Okay, go ahead and make whatever adjustments you want even if it is the one you always make. It's okay to do something just because you like it—as long as you are making a conscious choice and not being a slave to habit."

After a few breaths in this position, I ask them to take a rest by sitting down on their cushions.

"At the same time that what we do on the mat can be considered practice for when we are off the mat, we are also living the practice right then and there. It's not the same as if we were knitting a sweater that we will wear later or making a cake that we will eat later. In yoga we are wearing the sweater at the same time that we are knitting it, and, yes, we are actually making our cake and eating it, too."

The studio has thirty-eight people sitting on cushions and yet it is so quiet. The space feels empty and full at the same time. The students are still and entirely engaged. I notice how I'm getting the benefit of the yoga goodness just from watching them; even their breathing practice makes me feel more centered. I think once again how brilliant yoga is.

———✦———

January is a good time to go to India. It's cool in the morning and the evening, and the hot middle hours are perfect for napping. There I was in Uttar Pradesh and it was true, I couldn't have cared less that my long brown hair had short gray roots. I felt relaxed and content, bouncing along miles of dirt roads in a rickety bus with Gelek Rimpoche and my fellow travelers, all good friends from my meditation group. I was almost glad that I had a wide, squishy bottom. At least it provided the comfort of a padded seat!

We were told that this region of India was the most poverty stricken and riddled with bandits and Maoists, who very likely might accost us so we kept moving as long as it was daylight. Through the bus windows, I watched people huddle together around the village radio or get their beards shaved in open-air barber shacks. Women led bony goats behind them on the dusty roads home, sometimes squatting on their haunches to chew some betel root or take a pee right out in the open. It wasn't just being in another country; it was like being in another century.

Each time we got off the bus, we were surrounded by begging mothers holding their babies in their arms and crippled lepers leaning on sticks selling Buddha tsotchkes. Everyone was poor and dirty and very thin. Barefoot children chased after us chanting, "Om Mani Padme Hum, No Money Go Home." That made us laugh but it was hard not to feel guilty about our affluence. We all bought the Ganesh medallions and wooden statues and the incense, but over time it also become hard not to be annoyed that they didn't seem to believe us when we said, "No, thank you. I do not want another Buddha sticker." We knew that these thin, dusty people were desperate and that we were their best hope for making some rupees that day.

Back on the bus, those uncomfortable thoughts were jostled away and I sat staring blankly at the vast Indian countryside. I watched women in red and gold and turquoise saris walking across the fields carrying vases on their heads. The saris blew in the breeze, making a poetic picture of elegance that belied the women's poverty. I looked at those pretty clothes and started to think about what I would wear to the dinner buffet that evening at one of the Lotus Nikko hotels along the pilgrimage route where we were staying.

Although I was dying for a drink, some chocolate, and a strong cup of Starbucks, I told myself it was just as well that the hotel vegetarian buffets did not offer anything fattening and rewarding. Rimpoche warned us against eating dairy or salad or any fruit that didn't come in its own jacket. No sugar, no dairy, no alcohol, no meat—hmmm . . . maybe I could lose some weight on this trip after all.

Unconsciously I slipped my hand under my jacket to feel my belly. Was it still round or was it getting a little bit flatter? Every day I would check out the lay of my body-land. It definitely felt like my thighs were getting wider from sitting on this bus for so many hours. I gave myself a site-appropriate version of a familiar pep talk: "I'm going to be more disciplined with exercise on our fifteen-minute breaks. Too many snakes and piles of shit for sit-ups in the grass but maybe I can jog around the parking lot." I was hoping I could wear my new elegant Indian kurtas from FabIndia when I got back to the U.S. And I was hoping . . . what?

As I was squishing my belly fat in my hand and thinking about how much I hated my stomach and my wobbly butt, I suddenly realized how insane that was. Here I was, surrounded by people who were so thin that they regarded fatness as a sign of success and health. The children were thin. The police were thin. The hotel waiters were thin. Even the oxen were thin. And here I was hating my body and obsessing about my tummy roll and what I was going to wear as I schlepped through the dusty streets of India on a spiritual quest!

It took a few days for me to put two and two together, but eventually I recognized a certain ironic resonance between my inner drama and what the Buddha himself had experienced. Born into a royal family, given the name Gautama, and raised by a loving family and many servants in a luxurious palace, in his youth the Buddha had been showered with every privilege and sheltered from the harsh realities of the outside world.

As you might expect if you have a teenager, eventually he got bored. One night, when he was still a young man, Gautama snuck out of the palace grounds to have a look at the real world. What he saw shook him to his core. Instead of the beauty and lush comfort of his life in the palace, he saw people who were sick and suffering, others who were old and struggling to walk, and even a corpse. He had never seen the full spectrum of life and was both moved and confused. Soon after, he left his royal life and went out into the world to try to make sense of what he had seen.

The path that he walked was the same journey that our bus was following, twenty-six hundred years later. We visited the palace grounds and ruins and walked out the East Gate just as Gautama did when he went on his own pilgrimage to find truth. After leaving the palace, the young prince met others who were on a similar quest for understanding. Like me, he began by studying and practicing yoga.

I'd read in Karen Armstrong's book *Buddha* that Gautama actually practiced many of the same yoga postures and breathing exercises that I teach my students today, which I thought was pretty cool. By all accounts, he became the most accomplished yogi around, so motivated by his desire to be the master of his body that he surpassed all his teachers.

Eventually Gautama joined other extreme seekers who lived in the forest, engaging in punishing ascetic practices such as fasting, standing on one leg for many days, and threading needles through their tongues. These yogis believed that the source of all suffering is the body. After all, isn't the body the part of us that gets sick or injured, that grows old, dies, and ultimately dissolves? Isn't the body where desire comes from and doesn't desire lead to craving, which is the source of discontentment and unhappiness? The path to transcendence, they reasoned, must be total rejection of the physical body. Through self-abusive disciplines, they were trying to deny the impact of physical sensation and move beyond hunger and cold and pain. This was body hatred at its most elegant.

Here, too, Gautama excelled. He slept on nails and ate only nettles, turning green and becoming so thin his body was nearly all bones. Fortunately, a young woman named Sujata noticed Gautama as he was practicing in a bamboo grove beside the Niranjana River. Moved by his emaciated form, she offered him something to drink. Some say it was rice milk or lassi—a kind of smoothie that must have been very tempting out there in the parched Indian countryside. To the shock and disdain of his colleagues, Gautama drank it. I like that it took a woman to get the future Buddha to eat something.

The river where Gautama had been sitting when he accepted Sujata's gift was dried up on the day we visited. To get to the sacred site, we had to walk quite a ways along narrow elevated footpaths through rice paddy fields. Suddenly, out of nowhere, Chandra showed up. A thin young man who spoke English quite well, he became my guide and told me the story of Sujata and Gautama. He really was a first-class gentleman in secondhand clothes and it was nice holding his hand as he steadied me along the parts of the path that were crumbling away. I knew he would ask me for money at some point but I fell a little bit in love with him anyway. He told me he was in school and he liked practicing English and he clearly liked making new friends. He gave me his email address and asked me to be his pen pal. When we got to the actual site there wasn't much to see—a fire pit, a sacred tree—and I didn't think I was experiencing anything profound. But when I said good-bye to Chandra and got back on the bus, I burst into tears and cried for half an hour.

The story Chandra told me echoed in my mind. Fortified by the nourishment offered by Sujata, Gautama recognized that

torturing the body wasn't the way to relieve suffering, after all.
I can only imagine that he must have felt much better after having that drink, more clear-headed and physically energized.
Though he had tried to make himself immune to pain by fasting and self-denial, he was starting to figure out that being
trapped in a cycle of extremes only leads to more confusion and
unhappiness. Though the story happened a long time ago, something about that body obsession and resentment felt immediate
and real to me.

———————

We left the dried-up river and rode to muddy Bodhgaya, the
town Gautama put on the map by getting enlightened there.
That place didn't feel extra sacred to me, either, with all the
cheesy colored lights and pushy pilgrims elbowing their way
into the nonstop flow of the crowd circumambulating the temple, until we were ushered to a private area reserved for high
lamas such as Gelek Rimpoche.

Rimpoche gathered us together in a quiet spot under the
massive branches of the fourth-generation Bodhi tree. We were
told this was the very spot that Gautama had chosen to sit
down, cross his legs in lotus position, and meditate. By now he
had figured out that freedom from suffering wouldn't come
from rejecting the body or rejecting any part of himself. Gautama was committed to staying under the tree for as long as it
took to understand the true source of happiness.

Rimpoche told us that for forty days and nights, Gautama
meditated under the Bodhi tree. Eventually he had a powerful

realization that all the obstacles he ever experienced were in his own mind. He realized that thoughts are not solid, which means they can be changed. He discovered how to let go of the thoughts that generate fear, aggression, and hatred and how to transform that energy into love and compassion.

Armed with this new and profound understanding, Gautama stood up and walked away from the tree, into the forest. He ran into his old colleagues, who immediately recognized Gautama's fresh sense of clarity and wakefulness. They called him Buddha, which means the "one who is awake." They asked him to be their teacher. I could tell that this was all very real and alive for Rimpoche. I was moved to be sharing this experience with my own Buddhist teacher. As we left the sacred spot, I picked up two fallen Bodhi tree leaves and slid them between the pages in my dharma notebook.

By the time we had traveled to the next site, the one where Buddha gave his first teaching, I had a respiratory infection from breathing in the polluted air and cremation smoke near the Ganges. Stuffing some tissues in my pockets, I schlepped to the restaurant where our group was having lunch. I sat with my feet tucked under me because I don't particularly like having mice run over my toes while I'm eating. The night before we'd stayed at the Varanasi Radisson, a real hotel with real food, which was a nice change for us pilgrims. I promptly forgot that I was in India and had room service bring me my favorite meal of a chicken Caesar salad and red wine. Now I was curled up on a rickety folding chair with a drippy nose, an upset stomach, nervous toes, and a bad mood. I felt distinctly uninspired and unenlightened.

Then everything changed. After lunch, we entered the Deer

Park and saw Buddha and his first disciples sitting in a circle. They were actually statues, but life-size and painted with lifelike colors. You could see the drape of their saffron monk's robes flowing down their legs with their feet poking out. You could see individual strands of hair and fingernails on folded hands. As I looked at them, these beautiful statues did what statues some-times do—they threatened to come alive. And right then, I got it. Lightbulb flash! All this stuff we'd been studying, all these places we'd been visiting, it all really happened. Buddha was really a real person, just like you and me, only way more disciplined. I get the message, Rimpoche—if he could do it, we could do it, too.

My bad mood lifted and I felt buoyed by these precious teachings that Buddha gave at the Deer Park, which have been passed down in an unbroken lineage to my own teacher. I was filled with gratitude for all that I had learned from Rimpoche. It is said that the chance to meet the teachings of the Buddha in one's lifetime is as rare as the likelihood of a tortoise swimming in the vast ocean and just happening to pop its head up as an inner tube floats by.

We gathered around Rimpoche to hear that same first lesson that Buddha gave his colleagues-now-disciples.

"Everyone experiences discomfort. Even when you are just sitting still, doing nothing, you may still feel aches and pains. And even if you don't, if everything is fine right now, you may still recall past slights and get stuck in a bad memory, or find yourself experiencing fear of the future. When we relive the past and worry about the future, we miss out on our life." Rim-poche reminded us that in this way we are all alike—this is part of what it means to be human.

The good news is that once we recognize that we are creating our own discontentment we can change it. How do we do that?

When Gautama accepted the smoothie from Sujata, he took the first step away from the extremes of his own life—attachment to the lavish decadence of his royal home versus the intense aversion to all physical comfort—and toward a more healthy, more friendly middle path. Sweep the dust and sweep the dirt.

A famous Buddhist story, which illustrates this point, tells of a musician who asked the Buddha, "How should I practice?"

Buddha replied, "How do you tune your instrument?"

The musician answered, "Not too tight, not too loose."

The Buddha said, "Exactly like that."

My body has been my instrument for so long. I wondered if I could stop hating it once and for all. Could I apply this map for liberation to my own life? Sweep the dust and sweep the dirt. I wanted to find a middle path that was less dissonant, more harmonious, more in tune with what I've been teaching my students.

———— ◆ ————

The word *suffering* doesn't come up too often in yoga circles, but the word *sukha* gets bantered around a lot.

My students all know the pose called Sukhasana, or Easy Pose. Once again I throw them a pop quiz:

"Who knows what the word *sukha* means?"

"Easy."

"Space."

"A sense of ease."

The last answer reminds me of learning the sewing term *ease* in my high-school tailoring class. Our teacher taught us how to use a long, loose stitch to create a little bit of give in the shoulder seams of the formal white shirts she required us to make. Without that built-in "ease" or extra space in the shoulders, our sleeves would have ripped as soon as we tried to hug someone.

"*Sukha* doesn't exactly mean ease, but you're on the right track. The Sanskrit word *kha,* which means 'space' or 'sky,' was originally the word for 'hole.' Picture people riding in an ancient cart that rolls along on big wooden wheels. In the middle of the cartwheel is a large hole through which the axle is threaded. If the inside surface of the wooden hole had a smooth finish, the riders would have a comfortable ride. The prefix *su–* is translated as 'good,' as in wholesome, high, evolved, desirable, or even strong and stable. *Sukha* then refers to a good axle hole, but since we don't ride in oxen-drawn carts these days we can think of sukha as wholesome space.

"How many people are comfortable right now, sitting in Sukhasana? Who feels like they are in a wholesome space?"

I look around at the group. Most hands go up but not all. The pose is a basic cross-legged position, knees out to the sides with one ankle placed in front of the other. Everybody who practices yoga on even a semi-regular basis will be familiar with this pose. It is obvious to me which people like it, who hates it, who has a workable relationship with this pose, and who hopes we can go on to something else soon. I especially want to help the students in that last group.

"If your pelvis is tucking under or you aren't able to sit up tall or your back is hurting you in any way, please place at least two cushions under your seat. You'll notice right away that you can sit up with much less effort. Now put a yoga block underneath each knee so your legs can drop down to gravity without straining your inner thigh muscles. How does that feel?"

Most of the people who were uncomfortable before are nodding to let me know this is working well for them. But there are still a few who resist doing what I've suggested. They are so used to feeling the opposite of ease that they don't even know it could be different. I recognize that habit, too.

I haven't allowed myself enough ease—to grow or to move—either in my body or my mind. If my practice is about creating the causes and conditions for sukha to arise, I've been stuck doing just the opposite. Instead of allowing some looseness and give, I've habitually sewn narrow, unyielding stitches around my definition of a good female body. This tangled-up attitude toward myself is isolating and lonely. No wonder I can't find a way to hug myself, to embrace who I am, as I am, right now.

"The opposite of sukha is . . ."

"Dukha!"

"Right, which means . . . ?"

"Suffering?"

"Well, actually it means poor axle hole but that isn't really that relevant to us so, yeah, over the centuries it has been used to indicate suffering. If the inner perimeter of the hole were irregular or rough, if there were grooves or splinters inside, then with each turn of the wheel, the cart would jerk or thud. The riders would have a bumpy ride. You can imagine that this led to bruises and motion sickness and crabbiness among the passengers."

I can see that some of the students love this lesson, while others are getting uncomfortable and frustrated and bored. That's okay. Part of practice is not running away from discomfort but learning to work with it. In fact, that's exactly what this lesson is about.

"Okay, one more—what does *asana* mean?"

"Pose."

"Seat."

"Ground."

"It's a combo of all of the above. *Asana* means to sit with what comes up when you put your body is this particular shape. Our bodies are sort of like carts; they are the vehicles we live in as we move through the world."

There might have been some eye rolling at that corny metaphor but I bravely continue.

"My friend Enkyo Roshi talks about dukha through the example of a grocery cart. You know what she means, right? We've all gotten that cart with the wobbly wheel. You keep trying to straighten it out but it doesn't cooperate and there you are in the grocery store fighting with a full cart of groceries, getting mad and thinking, 'Why do I always get the lame cart?' "

Someone calls out, "Let's blame it on the cart!" And everybody gets a good laugh. I'm glad. A sense of humor is a key element of ease.

"You're right. Dukha is really not about the cart; it's more about the negative emotional disturbance that comes up in our mind when we feel like things are not fitting together. And it only gets worse when we start to feel like we get caught in that same situation over and over again.

"That's actually what we're practicing here in our asana class. We're consciously tying ourselves up in knots and then sitting with what-ever arises. If you stay steady, relax, and pay attention to what's hap-pening, then—theoretically—you can make skillful choices, right?

"So if your hips hurt in Sukhasana and you don't help yourself by sit-ting up on a cushion and creating some ease, well, then you're actually practicing Dukhasana! And, what's the point of that? We don't need to come to yoga to practice creating more suffering—we're already really good at that!" More smiles and it seems to have worked; there is definitely a more spacious vibe in the room.

———✦———

I like thinking about the people in the wooden cart, riding along the dirt roads full of potholes and muddy ruts. Just like my students, they would all have different ways of dealing with their bad axle-hole day. I imagine some of the people would curse with every jostle and others wouldn't even notice. There might even be some people who like the reliability of the bump; it might be uncomfortable but something about it is familiar and that is safe.

Both of these approaches are end games and I wonder about how the middle path relates to this. It's ironic, but integrating give and ease into any situation actually creates strength and stability. That's why I feel so destabilized right now. I'm starting to become aware that the seams I've habitually sewn to hold my life together may be too tight. I'd like to put my arms around myself but I'm afraid things will rip apart.

Walking down Broadway one night after yoga class, my friend Mary listened to me talk about how the practice of yoga helps people connect deeply with themselves and enables them to truly feel comfortable with who they are, as they are.

"So," she says, "does that mean you are a fraud?" That's why she's been my friend for so long. She knows me so well. And honestly, I've wondered that myself, although I remember someone wise telling me that all teachers feel like they are frauds.

Even though they are imaginary, I get inspired when I think that there would surely be a few jolly folk in the cart. These are the ones who, realizing the journey won't be forever, get a little kick out of the whole *ker-plunk, ker-plunk, ker-plunk,* nodding to one another with each jagged turn of the wheel, "Yep, there it goes again." Riding on the bus in India was like that for me. I didn't mind the bumps and constant horn honking and near head-on collisions. The dukha I felt was coming from inside me.

Maybe up until that point I just wasn't hurting that badly. Or perhaps my years of practice were starting to make a difference. Either way, I could no longer ignore that grouchy inner voice that starting nagging whenever I felt defeated by my body. It said only nasty stuff like, "These pointy shoes are killing me!" "Why are my feet so big?" "I hate the way this hat looks on my head." "This belt is making my fat stomach squish out of this top." "Why can't I look good in this outfit?" The voice got espe-cially persistent and annoying whenever I got frustrated, which generally meant I was trying to make permanent something that by its nature is meant to change and evolve. And by something, I mean me.

———◆———

Having gray hair might be one of the ingredients that created the causes and conditions for some new awakenings after return-ing home from India. Every day I meet a woman who tells me how much she loves my gray hair and how much she wants to let her own hair go gray. She says that she thinks I am so brave but she is not yet ready to be that brave. But having gray hair doesn't feel brave to me. What it feels is good and liberating and natural and healthy in so many ways.

I'm no longer strengthening the imprints that tell me I'm wrong or need improvement—at least in my hair department. That might not seem like a big deal but it is. Those old neurological synapses with the grouchy inner voice have dissolved and new ones have formed around positive feelings toward my silver locks. It might not seem like a big deal and in the grand scheme of suffering, it is a Cadillac problem. But for me it was a significant step toward self-acceptance, and in that way, I guess it was brave.

That little bit of motivation started turning my thought wheels in the opposite direction. I remembered what my meditation teacher told me, that being kind to others has to start with being kind to ourselves. And isn't that the very first teaching of yoga, ahimsa, which means non-harming of self and others? How could I turn this thing around?

One day, a few months after arriving home from India, full of my habitual frustration, discontent, and grumpiness about my body, a space opened up in the thicket of mental brambles and this thought floated in: "You already have everything you need to be happy."

Bingo! All of us experience moments of insight that pop up out of nowhere. Maybe it was a matter of time and practice . . . *drip, drip, drip,* the bucket fills. Or maybe something more ordinary like boredom or exhaustion or jet lag slows us down long enough to notice.

What I wanted had been there all along, but I was too busy creating my own dukha to notice it. I see that tendency in my students, too. They might be sitting nicely in a pose but the space between their eyebrows has a deep crease that tells me they are in pain. When I ask them about it, it's almost like I woke them out of a nap. A typical reply might be, "Oh yeah, this position always kills me. It's been like that for years. I just don't have good shoulders."

When I suggest that they loosen their grasp and use a yoga belt to allow the position to be held with less stress on their shoulders, it comes as a huge revelation! What a good idea. Here's a way to do the same thing without struggling and I could have been doing it that way all along. And, by the way, there's nothing wrong with your shoulders!

That day, in the snap of a finger, I saw that I had gotten it wrong all these years! I was always getting mad at my body but, in fact, my body has been fine. It's my relationship to my body that is hurting me, and my mind that is the real troublemaker. The truth is, although I've always had a perfectly fine, healthy body, I have thought and felt that I was too fat or too soft or too thin or too little here or too big there every day of my life. Simply put, I am addicted to hating my body and, really, to hating myself.

Clearly, it's my mind that needs to change, not my body. Instead of looking outside myself for a better diet, a more effective exercise plan, a face lift in a bottle, or an ultra-enthusiastic bra, I needed to examine my habitual ways of thinking—this addiction that has so defined my own self-image. I began to wonder who I would be without it. The first step to finding the answer to that question was to take a closer look at the problem.

What's the real reason I hate my body? I'm starting to understand that I've been basing my happiness on a specific condition, a condition that is not only impossible to achieve but is also a moving target. Like all forms of conditional happiness—more chocolate, shopping, money, alcohol—running after a "perfect" body can only result in hamster wheels of confused, desperate, and repetitive activity. Just like any other form of craving, there is no end to it, and no lasting satisfaction is possible.

This insight had been trying to get my attention for a while. Just like yoga students who stay in a position for years without even noticing, I hadn't even realized I was miserable but now that I did, I saw how long I'd been this way. I saw all the ways that I had tried to feel better by changing my body, looking everywhere for answers except for inside my head.

———•◆•———

Does any of this feel familiar? I know I'm not the only one who has been living with a hardhearted attitude toward herself. I know this because I hear it every day from my female yoga students. When they are not on the yoga mat, these smart women happen to be busy working as corporate executives and college professors and magazine editors and clothing designers and retail shop owners and app inventors and personal assistants and athletes and chefs and grandmothers.

These students ask me for advice about their bodies and their confidence, as if—because I am a yoga teacher—I know a secret they don't know. Well, the one thing I know for sure is, at this point, I've tried everything. I went to a chiropractor/nutritionist who tried to sell me a giant tin of protein powder, and then while I was facedown on the table, she asked me if I would hire her to teach a workshop at my yoga studio. I had a consultation with an Ayurvedic doctor who told me to chant "RAM RAM RAM" all day and then gave me some orange powder to eat that made my skin so hot I had to go home and lie naked on my bed with the air conditioner on full blast. I called him to see if that was what was supposed to happen, but he never returned my call.

I'd even bulked up while teaching Sweet and Low, my low-impact aerobics class, and Sweat Like Hell, my special gym dance class with hand weights and ankle weights. These classes were packed every night. Most of the other teachers at Crunch wore belly-baring, short-short outfits and I'm sure many students were drawn to them because they wanted to look that good, too.

That was not the case with my classes. I often had students who were thinner and more buff than me, but my classes were sold out because I taught a great workout and knew how to have fun. Every exercise had a name, and after a while, I started to put them down on paper in a book called *Sweat Like Hell, or A Girls' Guide to Perky Boobs*. The book was an exercise program, but even then I started it by encouraging readers to take a moment to acknowledge what they liked about their bodies: their thick luscious hair or their creamy skin or elegant collarbones. Here is a quote from the chapter called "It's My Mother's Fault."

Another phenomena handed down from mothers to daughters is cel-lulite. Many women have cellulite. Why is it that it's not thought of as a sexy, womanly thing like round hips or soft breasts? That's what I really want to know. Because I feel like hating cellulite is just another way that women have been taught to hate themselves. You know the routine: Monday I hate my stomach; Tuesday I hate my thighs; Wednesday my arms; Thursday my butt; Friday my butt even more; Saturday I hate my whole body; and Sunday I hate myself for hating myself.

But here's the good news. It turns out that men don't really even notice cellulite. I told my girlfriend that and she came to the conclusion that guys have gotten so used to seeing cellulite on all the women they've been with that they just think it's normal. That makes sense, right? Just like we are used to seeing a round squishy thing on the front of their bodies. No, not that thing. I mean their belly, gut, spare tire, which we accept as normal and love them anyway.

I go on to remind readers that we can't change our DNA, suggesting that "We don't really want to be somebody else. We just want to be more deeply fabulously ourselves." Too bad I didn't take my own advice, as usual.

Then I follow this self-help pep talk speak with exercises specifically designed as solutions to the target areas we blame for our discontent.

✦ The Schwahanga—leg lifts that firm up the outer upper thigh (sometimes called saddle bags, but I liked the word *schwahanga* because that is the sound they make when you walk).

✦ The John F. Kennedy President's Fitness Club of America—also known as V-sits. It turned out I wasn't the only one in the classes who first did this kind of sit-up in 1965 as part of JFK's fitness plan for America. I learned them from my seventh grade gym teacher who had us lifting our legs and our backs up to a 45-degree angle, turning our bodies into human V shapes. We did our JFK fitness routine to the Beach Boys' hit *California Girls*, and when it got to the part about the Northern girls keeping their boyfriends warm at night, we Seattle girls would pop up into the V-Sit and get semi–turned on, proud that we could keep boys warm at night even though I, for one, had no idea what that might entail.

✦   The International Grandmother's Exercise targeted upper arm flab; The Slut with Good Alignment toned the inner thighs; The Superwoman firmed up the back muscles; and then, of course, there was the Perky Boob Series.

One of the most detailed exercise solutions was the Party Position, which began with a description of the topography of the butt.

The Butt Map

✦   Butt Proper: The peak or summit of the butt

✦   Butt Waist: Where the two meet

✦   Leg Butt: She Whose Name Must Not Be Spoken

✦   Side Butt: Should be your side but instead it's more butt

✦   Side Leg Butt: aka The Schwahangas

✦   Side Butt Waist: More commonly referred to as Love Handles on men's bodies but called "no waist whatsoever" on women.

You get the idea. Although I thought I was being positive and encouraging, unconsciously I was working off the Joan Rivers/Phyllis Diller model of always making fun of your body, not realizing that is one of the most insidious methods for promoting low self-esteem.

My boyfriend at the time made a copy of *A Girls' Guide to Perky Boobs* and gave it to a literary agent, a friend of his that he hoped might give me some advice or even want to represent the book. The agent hated the book and said it wasn't funny. And in the end, he was right. It might have been a cute and fun way to get through your exercise routine, but, at the same time, it planted pretty mean seeds. Maybe it was just that very thinking that prevented my body from being how I wanted it to be, because even teaching lots of exercise classes didn't get me the results I wanted for more than a minute.

My students also ask me what they should eat. I never want to tell them because I know each person has a different makeup and we should each have different diets. Not only that, but as life changes, our diet should change, too, right? Based on that theory, over the years I have tried a wide range of diet explorations: macrobiotic, vegetarian, fruit juice fasts, food journals, calorie counting, fat gram counting, no cheese, no wheat, no sugar, no eggs, more protein, more sparkling water, much too much celery, and the completely unsuccessful mindful-eating diet based on the notion that if you paid attention to what you eat, you'd eat only good things in appropriate quantities. Further experiments in fasting, cleansing, colonics, saunas, and detox teas rounded out my quest for reliable digestion and smooth thighs, because, no, I didn't feel okay about my cellulite.

But mostly I ate like a normal person. I've never been drastically overweight and I've never been drastically underweight. I've never had a food addiction or an eating disorder. I exercise regularly but I'm not a gym junkie or a body builder. I'm a normal-sized woman with a normal-shaped body. And the other thing that seems to be very normal about me is that my opinion of my body is out of touch with reality and out of balance with what else I could spend my time on.

My friend Jeni told me she has always felt like she was fat, too. In fact, her father used to berate her and physically beat her for being overweight. She grew up believing that her weight was a strike against her, even influencing whether people liked her. Now Jeni is forty-nine and she likes her body. She has figured out how to be the weight she wants. She is married to a nice man and has two children. Her life isn't perfect and she isn't happy about everything, but it's not bad.

Recently Jeni and her husband, Dan, took a trip to Israel. Years before they met, Jeni had lived there and she wanted to introduce Dan to her old stomping grounds and her old friends, including her former fiancé, Ari. Jeni felt good about being married to such a great guy, but still it was nervous-making to see

Ari, especially since he was the one who broke off the engagement. The good part was that she suspected he had ended the relationship because he didn't like how fat she had been back then. Now that she was in good shape she no longer felt ashamed about her body. Even though she was shy about seeing Ari, she felt a certain level of confidence from knowing that she wasn't fat anymore.

As soon as they all met up, Ari's new girlfriend whispered loudly to him, "I thought you said she was fat!" She probably didn't care that her stage whisper was loud enough for Jeni to hear because she didn't know that Jeni understood Hebrew! So! Jeni's suspicions were confirmed—Ari had broken off the relationship because of her weight.

Later that day, Jeni and Ari took a walk together, just the two of them. He told her it was great to see her and that he was glad she was happy. He said, "I always knew you would leave Israel and go to live in America. That is why I broke up with you. I didn't want to leave Israel. Anyway," he said, "I wouldn't want to marry you now. You're much too thin."

Jeni was shocked to find out that Ari preferred a little bit of juiciness in his women. Like me, she had a tightly frozen idea of what was a good and desirable body. It never occurred to her that the idea she had about how she should look was not the same as Ari's. She managed to finally change her body into what she wanted only to discover it didn't match his idea of an attractive female figure at all. This gave her second thoughts about her suffering and her efforts. Was it worth it? Who was she trying to please anyway?

It seems that it's not just bodies that change; even our ideas about bodies change. I learned this at my mother's waist, literally. As a little girl, I would look up at my mom from the perfect vantage point of her waist, and observe the work required for her to get dressed up. I watched her hold the top of her side zipper with one hand, and then carefully tucking her luscious fleshiness into the side seam, she started zipping up. She held her breath so she wouldn't pinch her skin as she squeezed into the blue brocade satin dress she'd made for herself. Just like the ones that Elizabeth Taylor wore, it had a bosomy, tight bodice; a tiny, unforgiving waist; and a slim skirt that hugged her generous hips and thighs. What an hourglass! Stuffed into her ultra-feminine cocktail dress, I thought my mom was the most beautiful woman in the world, and so did my dad. My mom, on the other hand, probably couldn't breathe and certainly couldn't eat anything, but she had the fifties look down pat: velvety skin and soft arms with no muscle definition in sight. A woman was meant to be pliant and squishy, not hard and tight like a man or, heaven forbid, athletic, which was code for "lesbian," which was code for "non-feminine."

Those days are long gone. The trendy shape for bodies changes all the time but my mom never really changed that much. She got heavier as she got older and was always on a diet in the hopes of getting back to that hourglass body of her sexy thirty-something years. And I wonder, am I stuck in a time warp, too? Just as David and I noticed in our GA research that the worst-looking gray hairdos were the shags from the seventies that had never been updated, could it be that ideas about what shape is physically attractive can also become stuck in the past?

———•◆•———

Collette was in the pedicure chair next to me, and her long, wavy, glittering gray hair was so spectacular that I just had to ask her about it. Isn't it funny that now I am jealous of women who have hair that is more silver than mine? She told me she's never dyed it. When she had brown hair she never got compliments but now she always does. Collette has better things to do with her time than get her hair colored, and anyway she doesn't want the chemicals.

Collette had a confidence that I admired. Our talk about hair led to appearance led to bodies. She told me, "Women wax and wane naturally like the moon. We just haven't figured out that five pounds this way and that is not worthy of drama."

Collette has a sixty-year-old musician friend who'd always had flaming red hair—at first naturally and then with assistance. After some years, inspired by Colette, she finally cut her hair as short as she could stand in order to let the gray grow in; the same method I'd used. Two years later, she recorded a new album but when she saw the cover she started crying.

"Why?" asked Collette. "Is the music no good?"

"No, I just can't believe how old I look."

That same afternoon, Collette's thirteen-year-old daughter came home and asked her why the super skinny girls with big boobs are the most popular. "Well," Collette answered, "it depends on why you want to be popular." Her voice got quieter as she told me that this was new. Her daughter and all her friends, suddenly, just in that month, had decided that they are all fat.

Collette went to bed that night with a heavy heart, in between her sixty-year-old friend who feels old and her thirteen-year-old daughter who feels fat.

I never saw Collette again but I've thought of her so many times. Just as I want to help my students feel ease in their lives, I had that same impulse to ease her heart, too. Not only do I feel that impulse, but I've actually taken a vow to do that very thing.

———— ◆ ————

Twenty-five people on their best behavior are sitting on the floor in a misshapen circle. It's misshapen because nobody wants to sit right next to me. They're scared of me. Not because I'm scary, really, but because they don't know me yet. When they look at me, they think, "I'll have what she's having." They want to be a yoga teacher like me and that desire is so strong that they get intimidated by my very presence.

Of course, I know that and I also know it's a temporary phenomenon. We will all get to know one another very well as this four-month OM yoga Teacher Training program unfolds. Everyone in the circle has just told us their names, shared their yoga backgrounds and, at my request, tried to articulate why they want to take this yoga teacher training.

"I'm a sixth-grade teacher and I want to teach yoga to my kids."

"My anxiety attacks went away since I started yoga."

"My dance career is ending and vinyasa yoga satisfies my movement jones."

"I can't stand working as a lawyer one more day!"

My heart feels soft and open to each one of them as they bravely start sharing their stories. I make an effort to let them know that they have been seen and heard by me by doing my yoga class party trick. My eyes go around the circle again while I repeat each person's name. A couple times I hesitate and have to rummage around in my memory. It's a shared moment of suspense . . . Will she get that person's name? The student in question waits and I can see that he or she will feel bad if I don't remember the correct name, and I manage to pull it up. It's New York so the names run the gamut from Yuki to Ishmael to Renate, Parker, Peyton, and Luke.

Now there are only three people left and . . . oooh . . . What was her name? Aha! I remembered it and the next one and the next one and I did it! A round of applause as I laugh and say, "It's because of the headstand! Headstands develop mental clarity!" I laugh again and they do, too. My good memory is a victory for all of us; the first real bonding moment. But the truth is, it's not just the headstand that helps me here; it's my bodhisattva commitment. I am always looking for ways to help them feel acknowledged, especially important in this first meeting. I want them to feel happy and safe right away.

"Again, I welcome you all to OM yoga Teacher Training. We will get to the poses soon enough, but let's lay the groundwork for being here in the first place. The name of this training program is Joining Heaven and Earth. Has anyone been curious about that title?"

Still feeling shy, a couple of them nod but most just sit and wait for what I have to say next. "Heaven means your vision. Each one of you has a passion for yoga that has developed into a vision of sharing your beautiful practice with others. Am I right?" More nods.

"When you are imagining your future or how you would like your world to be, you might find yourself looking up at the clouds; that's heaven. The opposite of that is the grounding quality of earth, which is about making things happen now.

"It's wonderful to have a positive goal but without earth, it remains just a dream in your head. On the other hand, if you only have earth and no heaven, you might be good at tasks, like fixing the sink, but that will never evolve into a long-term goal or big vision: perhaps starting a plumbing business or inventing a better pipe. To be balanced, whole and effective, earth needs the vision of heaven and heaven needs the action of earth.

"Humans are the only beings who can bring heaven and earth together and you've already started doing that by showing up here today. You had an idea of being a yoga teacher and then you took steps toward that goal by filling out your application, sending in your money, keeping up your yoga practice, and showing up here today—on time, in appropriate clothing, with all your textbooks. Congratulations!"

Some of them are already taking notes and feeling inspired by this talk, which is relaxing them and helping them lose their self-consciousness.

"Now I have one more question for you: What is the reason for becoming a yoga teacher?"

They look up from their notebooks with blank stares.

"Okay, I'll give you a hint. It's not to get famous." I know some of them think I'm famous because I write for *Yoga Journal* and teach at many international yoga conferences. But that's a pretty small pool for fame. So I tell them about how I recently attended a Halloween party dressed as the great yoga master B. K. S. Iyengar. With fierce cotton eyebrows, the red line of a Brahmin dividing my forehead and a Nehru jacket, I thought my costume was obvious, but at that non-yoga party, the getup was a flop because not one person had ever heard of Mr. Iyengar. So, no, it's not about getting famous.

"And it's definitely not to get rich!" I know some of them think I'm rich because I have a big, beautiful yoga studio but that's just because they don't know how much it costs to run a business in New York City.

"So, what is the reason to be a yoga teacher? Some of you have already said it . . ."

"To help."

"Yes! That's right. The only reason to be a yoga teacher is to be helpful. That's the whole gig, and you know what? Sometimes it can be challenging! There will be people who come to your class who don't want to do what you ask them. Some have attitudes. Some people even have B.O. And sometimes a person comes to your class that you just don't like. But here they are. They have come to your class to learn yoga and find a sense of balance and well-being and your job is to help them. All of them, without exception.

"That's why I consider teaching to be a practice, just like doing yoga is a practice and meditating is a practice. But when I am practicing yoga on my mat, I'm doing it for myself . . . and that's the difference. The practice of teaching is really to benefit others and so we can think of teaching yoga as a bodhisattva practice. Does anyone know what *bodhisattva* means?"

Silence. Most of them are still too shy to answer and I'm pretty sure none of them are familiar with this word. Yoga teachings don't typically include this concept, so I backtrack to something they might have heard in a yoga class.

"Okay, does anyone know what the word *ahimsa* means?"

Hands fly up. I call on Luke, who is pleased that I still remember his name.

"Nonviolence?"

"Yes, non-harming of self and others. This is the bottom line of yoga practice, the very first principle. And did you notice that ahimsa is a 'non–,' a renunciation? That is where we start: from a place of not wanting to ever harm any living being. Then if we water that notion, like a flower, our heart opens and our motivation starts to blossom outward, shifting from non-doing to doing. Non-harming evolves into a purposeful activity of being helpful, and suddenly we see so many opportunities. When we have that feeling, it is like waking up to life a little bit, right?"

A few of the students are restless. They're not ready for this level of understanding yet; they want to get up and do some Sun Salutations. But most of the teacher trainees are on the edge of their cushions, knees tucked under their chests listening to me as if they were being read a great novel. They know this is the juice, this is the inside scoop on teaching right from the horse's mouth and they are drinking it up. They've stacked up yoga blocks to make desks on the floor and they're furiously taking notes.

I try to wake up the spaced-out people with a playful threat: "You should all be taking notes. You will actually be tested on this." I pause to let them all get organized for the big reveal.

"*Bodhi* means 'awakened,' and *sattva* means 'existence.' So *bodhisattva* means . . ."

Yuki blurts out, "Awakened life!"

"Yes! A bodhisattva is a person who is so awake in the world that they see the suffering of others. They dedicate their entire life to relieving this condition. Doesn't that sound like a good aspiration for a yoga teacher?"

I can tell that they like learning new exotic words like *bodhisattva* but they are also getting freaked out. I reassure them.

"Don't worry. You don't have to be a Buddhist to be a yoga teacher and you don't have to take a special bodhisattva vow to participate in this course but I offer you this model as an inspiration. A bodhisattva does what it takes to be helpful to all beings everywhere, all the time, no matter what.

"Different people learn in different ways: hearing, visuals, reading, touching, and doing. So you are here to develop your language, your hands-on adjustments, your voice, your eyes, your understanding of people, and your compassion. Because when a student doesn't understand what you are trying to teach, the bodhisattva says, 'I will dig deeper into my tool bag to find a way to communicate and help this person.' We are not really teaching poses; we are teaching and reaching people. And this is what it means to be a yoga teacher."

The room goes silent. The students are contemplating this, trying to put the pieces together. Others are clearly moved. In the gap, I realize how much this all means to me. Sandwiched between my students and my own dear teachers, I experience a feeling of warmth and gratitude.

Remembering that, like the tortoise in the ocean finding an inner tube, it is a rare opportunity to meet these precious teachings in one's lifetime, I inwardly recommit to the bodhisattva path. Not just as a yoga teacher, but in every moment, I vow to be helpful to every being I encounter in my life—all those beings I know and love, those I know and don't like so much, and all those many, many beings I'll never even meet.

During a recent dinner at the ultra-hip Bowery Hotel restaurant, our friends Mary and Allen asked if I was writing anything new. Popping a Parmesan-stuffed olive into my mouth, I said, "Yes, but the subject is top secret." Unable to resist that tantalizing tidbit, they begged me to let them guess. I sipped my Gavi while Allen, a genius inventor, tried to guess. "Is it about space?" "Is it about global warming?" David and I chuckled knowingly because it was clear that as smart as he was, Allen was never going to guess that I was writing a book about how women hate their bodies. Then Mary said, "Is it about women and bodies?" She smiled like a Cheshire cat as I quickly passed her the onion foccacia.

Mary and I have been complaining to each other about our bodies since we were naturally slim twenty-somethings with unwrinkled knees. Now that we are fifty-somethings, it is safe to say that we have become even more obsessed and distressed about our bodies. To say the least, we do not like to be naked with the lights on anymore. Not that we ever did.

This seems normal to me. But just because something is normal doesn't mean it is a good way to live.

I've spent my entire life working with my body and I enthusiastically advocate fitness and healthy eating. But having firm abs has not brought me joy. And you know what? I'm sick of it! I'm sick of feeling bad about myself because my body does not match an external notion of perfection.

Now that I see this syndrome in myself I see it everywhere.

And I feel sad about it. I feel sad about Collette and her daughter and her friend.

I feel sad about Jeni and all the men everywhere who can't convince their women that they are beautiful.

I feel sad for all the women who are playing the broken record that says, "I don't have the body I want and I don't want the body I have."

I feel a little less sad about my friend Jane, because at least she has a good sense of humor about it all. She told me she is going to create a yoga class called Yoga for When You Are Feeling Fat and I have no doubt it will be a huge success!

I feel sad about the women who tell me they are sick of dyeing their hair but they don't think they are brave enough to stop.

It took only an instant for me to feel bad about myself when I first saw my gray roots but it took a year to transform those feelings into something positive. My long gray hair flows beautifully around my shoulders and reminds me of the untangling of imprints that had to happen for me to be able to say, "I'm way less of a fraud now, Mary."

As a yoga teacher I know that ultimately the best way to give a good lesson is by manifesting it with full radiance. I feel sure that if I can apply the principles of meditation and yoga to my addiction to hating my body, things will begin to shift. Space will open up, appreciation will arise, and I'll probably get into a heck of a better mood.

If practice is supposed to be personal, if I really want to be a bodhisattva, if I really want to help others, I've got a golden opportunity here. So here goes:

I vow to stop trying to change my body and, instead, start to change my relationship to my body.

I vow to stop obsessing on losing weight and start focusing on losing self-aggression.

I vow to hold a healthy urge for self-improvement in my right hand and a strong sense of appreciation in my left hand and slowly, sensitively, bring my two hands together in a prayer that transforms *good enough* into *goodness*.

With a strong commitment it won't be hard because I know that basic goodness is already there, inside me all the time, if I just look in the mirror a little more closely.

I want to do this for my friend Mary, for all my students, and for every woman everywhere who is walking through life, accomplishing great things, giving to others, creating our world, and all the time hating her body because it's normal to do that.

This is the story about how everything I learned about my body was wrong. It is the story of how I lost trust in my own strong, clear arms and legs, the goodness of my curves, and the tenderness of my open heart. It's about how I gave up my power without even knowing I had it.

But it's also about how yoga and meditation gave me refuge, showed me a map, and reminded me that everything arises, abides, and dissolves. It's about how I recognized my own form of suffering and made a commitment to go for happiness instead. It's how I got off the bumpy bus and onto a path of ease. This is the story of me and my body and how we became friends again after so many years of fighting.

Well, anyway, I hope it is. But if I can see everything so clearly, why is that grumpy inner voice still whispering in my ear, planting hard thoughts in my mind? I've made progress but I think I need more medicine, bigger guns. It's time to get some help from those who have gone before me because I need some real tips, not the kind that cover up but the kind that cut through negativity and turn it into positivity. I've frozen the flow of this vinyasa long enough. I'm ready to plant new seeds.

Abiding

Abiding is an in-between experience. Because of that, it gets less attention. It's not a peak event such as arriving or departing or even an intentional action such as accumulating or releasing. Lacking obvious drama to pull you in, it is easy to miss or ignore or avoid.

But if you do place your attention on the liminal, allowing yourself to feel the threshold-space richness of neither here nor there, you discover that this is where the magic happens. It's when things start to cook.

A good yoga brew is made of the universal elements of heat and exertion, breath, sweaty muscles, and strong bones. In life, these same ingredients show up as tears and love, anger and fear, hope and confusion, sometimes nausea, sometimes heartbreak, sometimes joy.

The thing is, the alchemy only happens if you include everything. You can't leave out the dirty stuff that makes you antsy or scared or ashamed. It all goes into the pot, and then you watch and wait.

If you are impatient or pushy, the flavors won't blend properly, and you'll end up with clumps of unprocessed emotion. Sadness won't temper the anger, kindness won't quiet the boss of the brain, the fragrance of delight won't seduce the fear.

What do you get in the end? Nothing. Nothing solid, that is. Just a gut knowing that everything is really a 'tween, anyway. This knowing, which helps you stay the course no matter what, is the knowing that arises from abiding.

———— •◆•————

My mom takes her time pushing her rollator onto the industrial-sized elevator in her assisted-living home in Dallas. I bring up the rear. Possibly the slowest elevator in the world, there is enough time for a meaningful conversation between the lobby and my mom's apartment on the fourth floor. But naturally we slip into a variation of a conversation we've had my whole life.

Mom lifts her old lady hand off the handle of the walker, turns her palm up, and says, "Look," jiggling her forearm.

I say, "What?"

"I hate it."

"Hate what?"

"My wrinkly arm. I hate it."

Sigh. "You look great, Mom. And your outfit is adorable. You know they call you the best-dressed lady in the whole place!"

She smiled at that, but immediately got distracted by the mirrored elevator doors and began fidgeting with her Audrey Hepburn haircut that shows off her high cheekbones.

At eighty-three, my mom is still concerned with her looks, constantly fussing with her lipstick and necklace and always wanting to buy new clothes that are more flattering. Today she is wearing a pair of slim-fitting Eileen Fisher capris and a black-and-white-striped T-shirt sparkling with black rhinestones. She really is adorable. Even though she's not very steady on her feet, we still figured out a way for her to have attractive footwear. No old lady clunkers for her; I bought her pretty patent leather ballet flats with one little strap to hold her ankles tight. She needs that strap because we had to buy a bigger size after she had one big toenail removed. The other one is half fallen off, but even so she still likes to get ballet pink—and sometimes bubble-gum pink—pedicures.

My very feminine mom did a good job of teaching me how to be ladylike and strong at the same time. Every Sunday morning she sat at the dining room table doing her nails while she prepared the lesson she would teach to her Sunday school class. Her hands are so wobbly now that it's hard to believe how dexterous she once was. One of her most magical skills was that she could make a sewing knot with one hand just by manipulating the thread between her thumb and index finger. She showed me how to do it many times but I literally couldn't even see what happened, it went so fast. My attempts always resulted in a tangled mess of loose thread. Millie would laugh at my frustration and then show me again. Pulling a length of thread off the little spool, she would cut it with her teeth. Then holding the thread in one hand, she'd say, "Just go like this," and her thumb would swoosh a circle over her index finger, "and this," and there was the knot. She was showing off a little bit when she did this and I liked that part of my mom, too. The part that felt good about being able to do something slick and hyper-facile.

The strong things she taught me were fun, too. She showed me how to turn cartwheels on the beach, leaving sandy marks—handprint, handprint, footprint, footprint—in a straight line. She sang "Hey, Look Me Over" in the car to keep my spirits up on the way to the doctor. With my leg full of those fifty-six stitches, she egged me on until I joined in on the last line, "Hey, look out, world, here I come!" Like many moms, she was rarely ever sick.

Maybe that is why I didn't recognize something was seriously wrong when Millie started falling down. Or maybe I just didn't want to admit it. First, she sprained her ankle walking down the church steps, and then she fell and broke her arm in the Whole Foods parking lot. The worst was when she tripped over a door sill while carrying plates from the table and fell flat on her face, humiliated that she couldn't even manage that simple task and mortified that she'd broken all the plates.

It wasn't until years later after she'd been diagnosed with Parkinson's that we recognized this pattern and knew that she hadn't been spaced out or clumsy; she'd been getting sick. The heartbreaking part was how she would cry out, "I hate myself," every time she fell down. Not knowing a sickness had been growing in her, Millie assumed that falling was her fault, that she was uncoordinated, ungraceful, out of control, that she had ruined the evening for everyone. And that made her hate herself.

Shortly afterward, everything changed. The doorman at her apartment told me she went out shopping one morning, and when she came back, her head had dropped down to her chest. My phone started ringing with reports of her growing confusion, and when the manager of her apartment building called to tell me that Millie was wandering the hallways at midnight looking for my father (who had died several years earlier), I jumped on a plane and rushed to Dallas.

Now we know that my mom has Lewy body disease, which presents as a cruel combination of Alzheimer's and Parkinson's. The tremors in her hands, feet, and neck are causing her to collapse sideways into herself, as if she were starting to fold up in readiness for being put away for keeps. She has had a series of mini-strokes, which, according to her neurologist, have left Swiss cheese–like holes in her brain. That has created holes in her understanding of concepts like time and space, where and when, morning and night, days, weeks, hours. "Where are you?" she asks every time I call her from my home in Manhattan. "Oh, in New York? Can you come by for lunch today?"

My mom's interests have shrunk down to what she can handle and what matters to her, on a daily basis, whatever day or week it might be—and her primary interest is her appearance. If she can't feel good, at least she can do her best to look good. Even though her ankles are uncomfortably swollen and she is often cold, she mostly complains about her hairdo and how her clothes fit. I wonder about this. I'm not interested in blaming my mom for creating my body-loathing habits, because it's bigger than that. But now that I've started to recognize my own self-obsessive judging, I see it in her, too, and I wonder if I am genetically predisposed to this way of thinking.

Finally, back in her living room, I help my mom transfer from her walker to her recliner. This involves more physical intimacy than we've ever had in my memory. The Parkinson's creates cramping, so my first job is to pry her tightly curled fingers off the walker arms and place them onto my arms.

"Hold on to my wrists, Mom."

As she grapples for me, she loses her balance and starts to cry.

"No, no, we're not falling! It's okay. Hold on to me, Mom."

I manage to swing my body under hers just in time to stop her downward momentum. I'd rather have her tumble onto me than onto the floor. Please, don't let her get any more black eyes or purple bruises. My husband says I am literally carrying my mom on my back these days, and it's true. She appears frail but her dead weight is heavy and I've started having low back pain, which I know is not caused simply by the physical work involved in caring for my mom. But it's okay. She carried me when I was a baby, and now it's my turn to carry her.

We get upright again and start over. I lean back as if I were water-skiing to counterbalance her weight as I slowly lower her onto the maroon corduroy recliner. This time I've got a firm hold of her forearms; except for a bit more give in the skin, they feel just like my own arms. Another inch to go and she's down. *Plop.* We made it. I'm pleased, but Millie has a weird intense look on her face.

"What's the matter, Mom? Is something hurting you?"

"There's a bug."

"A bug?" I follow her gaze. "I don't see a bug."

"It's there on the carpet. It's been there for weeks."

Lewy body gives you hallucinations. She sees bugs on the carpet and holes in her closet floor and she hears invisible children playing in the hallway at night.

"I don't think there's a bug there today, Mom. It just looks like that sometimes because of the way your wheels flattened the carpet."

She doesn't really believe me, but she's willing to humor me and lets it go for now.

I slide the walker underneath my seat and perch there. Time to distract Millie. Reaching forward, I extend my hands to her, palms up. "Let's do some yoga." She never wants to do yoga, never has, never will. But she smiles anyway because she loves me and it's fun to do things together. When I'm not here she is stuck in this chair alone for hours. She takes my hands.

"Inhale," I say in my yoga teacher voice, lifting her arms up.

"Exhale," and I lower her arms.

"Inhale, exhale." I repeat these instructions on a lilt, my voice going up on the inhale and down on the exhale, to indicate her arms should do the same thing. Millie's arms don't go up very far, only about halfway up to shoulder height, but any movement is good for her. We do this four times, and then I alternate, taking her right arm up and down four times, and then her left arm up and down.

She follows my instructions, breathing in and out, and seems to be fully engaged. To me, this is a completely manifested vinyasa yoga practice. A common misconception about vinyasa yoga is that it is a kick-butt, super-sweaty form of yoga that can only be done by hard-core athletic yogis. But Millie is matching her breath to her movements and paying attention to the entire experience, not just the up position or down position, but the path all along the way. And now she is done and I'm tired, too.

I slide off the walker, kneel on the floor beside her, and open the box of family photos, getting ready for another familiar conversation. We both get a kick out of the fact that my mom and her three sisters, Donnabelle, Betty, and Beverly, all look so much alike. And all the girl cousins—Kelly, Sherry, and me—look like one another and we each look like our moms. And the whole bunch of us looks like Grandma. There are variations on the theme, of course, depending on age, diet, exercise, hairstyle, and which families live in the city or the country, but the genetic inheritance is clear. We all have the same defined cheekbones, deep-set eyes, and squarish chins, and if you turn us around, we all have the same upside-down heart-shaped bottoms, too.

"I think you are the prettiest of all the sisters, Mom."

She smiles, eyes lighting up and cheekbones coming into view. "I always thought so." Somehow the way she says that isn't mean or arrogant. It is sweet, and I am glad my mom thinks she is pretty. It's so painful to hear her complain about her body, but in the meantime, she's already forgotten what we were talking about and wants to know if I can take her to get a manicure.

———— ✦ ————

After our manicure we went to dinner at Good Eats, a neighborhood place that nicely accommodates old folks and walkers, especially at five thirty P.M. As part of my research into how other women have dealt with the issue of body image, of personal perception and self-confidence, I'd decided to start with my mom. I remember my dad telling me that the very first time he saw my pretty mom with her shy smile, crossing a footbridge at the church summer camp, he decided right then he was going to marry her. But I'm not so sure that my mom always felt beautiful and I know she's struggled with her weight for my whole life. After moving into the assisted-living home, she lost almost thirty pounds but not in a good way. Depression can make you stop eating all together. She was picking at her plate now, because she likes chicken fried steak and she was managing to eat the tiny bites I'd cut for her.

After I told her a little bit about my dilemma, the whole body drama, always wanting it to be different and never being satisfied with my body as it is, I hoped she might have some advice. Or that at least we would have an interesting conversation. Miraculously, we've never really talked about this in any significant way, just always talked around it, as I've done in most of my female relationships, all of which have been based on an unspoken agreement that it's natural to be unsatisfied with our bodies/hair/face in some way. Millie appeared to be listening as she ate her mashed potatoes and white gravy.

"So what do you think about this, Mom?"

"If you are pretty and thin, you get more attention."

I tried to go further with this, asking how she felt about that, but she didn't respond to my question. What was I thinking? Of course her brain is no longer configured in a way that allows her to follow a train of thought. That conversation was over and I was left to ponder that one telling statement.

The next week I asked her neurologist about the chances that I will get the same disease she has; am I genetically predisposed to Lewy body? I guess it isn't good news because he didn't give me a straight answer, although he did give me some advice: "If you do aerobic exercise, you will cut your chances by fifty percent." That was some kind of answer, I guess, and I made a promise to myself to renew my lapsed gym membership and get back to working with Smith. In the meantime, I can't help but wonder as I watch her decline what will become of me.

———— • ◆ • ————

I step to the front of the studio and say, "Everyone, please sit in Vajrasana." The students know this pose and take a few moments to reorganize their postures. Because I have trained them this way, they include moving between poses and arranging their mats and yoga props in their mindfulness practice, acknowledging that the in-between moments are as important as the asanas themselves. They neatly fold the Mexican blankets they were sitting on and stack them at the end of their mats. I laugh as I tell them, "Based on what my high school bedroom looked like, my mother would be shocked to hear me say this, but 'Form Creates Space.'"

The form, or posture, called Vajrasana is very simple. The students kneel, fold their legs beneath them, and sit down with their hips over their heels. They know that if it hurts their knees, they can place a blanket under their shins or in the fold between their calves and thighs. They take their time to set this up with clarity so that they can feel balanced and at ease in this position. They do it this way because I've taught them to do it this way. It's a reminder that at their core is Basic Goodness. They sit quietly like peaceful warriors, their palms down on their thighs, faces open, eyes soft and steady.

"Who knows what Vajrasana means? This word is actually made of two words—*vajra* and *asana*. The Sanskrit word *asana* typically refers to yoga posture or pose. But a more literal translation is 'to sit down.' I also think of it as meaning 'to sit with what comes up when you put yourself in this particular neurological pattern, this precise energetic circuit.'" Sitting in this position is not complicated. All of my students can do it easily.

"*Vajra* means 'diamond' or 'thunderbolt.' When we sit like this, we are reminded of what about us is diamond-like, adamantine, indestructible. And that is what is deep inside all of us. It's called Basic Goodness. Everyone has it. You were born with it; it's your heritage and it can never be taken from you. When we start to connect to our own Basic Goodness, to really feel it, we then begin to recognize it in others. Because everyone—including your noisy neighbors and their yapping dog, that aggressive person on the subway this morning, your ex-husband, and anyone else who is on your shit list—everyone has Basic Goodness. Including you. The Thunderbolt is what happens to us when we have a sudden moment of clarity and awakening. Traditionally, that is called a 'Flash of Lightning in the Dark of Night' and this is what pulls us out of our thick mind soup and reminds us again: At our core we are made of Basic Goodness."

The students sit quietly throughout, although I see a few tears.

———— ✦ ————

My dog, Leroy, turns in a circle eight times, each one getting smaller until he finally spirals into the perfect position for a poop. When he finishes, he makes one more circle, and then because he feels so good now, so nice and light, he wags his tail and kick his legs in a Shave-and-a-Haircut-Six-Bits rhythm. This routine never varies. He never thinks, I'm just going to squat down here and go. Leroy is a very bright poodle, definitely the Einstein of the dog park. Yet he lives in a choice-less world, his behavior dictated by habit and the fact that he is a member of the animal realm.

People are animals, too, but we live in the human realm, a world full of options. The thing is that it's up to us to try something new. We all get stuck in Leroy-like ruts, but since we are humans, we have the ability to recognize and then shift things, theoretically.

So why do I still start off every morning by recycling this mental broken record: "Okay, last night I had two pieces of bread and one glass of wine and extra shavings of Parmesan on my Caesar salad. Why? Why did I do that? I feel so fat now. It's going to take me another whole day just to get back to non-bloatedness. Okay, today I'm going to do better. I'm going to have oatmeal with flax seeds and blueberries for breakfast and lunch will be a medium soup from Whole Foods and then if I really want to I can have a nonfat cappuccino in the afternoon. Ooh, what is that squishy bit over here—ugh. Maybe I'll go shopping and find something that makes me look good . . . or not. Shit, I'm so fat!"

Mark Bittman writes in *Food Matters* that eating food is not an addiction like cigarettes or coffee or alcohol. If you eat a little bit too much one night, it's no big deal. Just get back on your healthy program the next day and carry on. No guilt necessary. No drama necessary.

This is so hard for me to do. For as long as I can remember, I've been stuck in a circular animal-realm-thinking pattern that whispers, "It's your fault. Your body is out of whack, out of control. Whatever you are doing, eating, not eating is wrong. You can't control your body, it doesn't respond the way you want, and it's your fault."

What a double bind. Of course, in those moments when I'm thinking straight, I certainly agree with Mark Bittman that if you overeat one day you can modify the next and just get back on track and it's no big deal. But when you start thinking your body is something separate from you, logic goes out the window and things get complicated.

I remember the days when I used to eat whatever I wanted without a second thought. It was during my early college days in the seventies, which meant there was a lot of dope smoking going on, always followed by an irresistible case of the munch-ies. My buddy Terry and I knew the secret to satisfying the munchies was just the right balance of sweet (chocolate, choco-late, chocolate) and salty (Doritos). Lots of soda to wash it down. I realize now that this was how I trained myself to act and think. My philosophy then was if you have a craving, then do what you can, as quickly as you can, to satisfy it. I wasn't interested in curbing my urges, and if I was a slave to them, I wasn't that uncomfortable about it yet. Maybe that's denial, but I never once thought about changing that syndrome. Why should I? I was having fun and never gained one pound, even though Terry and I did obsess about the size and shape of our thighs.

Even then the drama was really the addiction. I'm hooked on the self-loathing, judgmental attitude that goes around and around in a circle, just like Leroy, telling me if I don't like the way I look, then I must be doing something wrong, or there is something wrong with me. Either way, I am a wrong person. This leaves me feeling helpless and hopeless.

This misguided thinking kicked into full gear when my nat-urally thin body started filling out in my early thirties. I had already developed a fear of fat and a fear of food. I had also developed a daily habit of starting the morning with a negative chant of regret, recrimination, and a vow to do better—a mil-lion variations on the above. Yet the changes I wanted never happened. What was I missing? I don't eat fried foods. I avoid gluten. I rarely eat dairy. I exercise pretty much every day and I haven't eaten red meat since 1971. Why have I gained weight every year for the last fifteen years? Hearing me complain about this, a yoga colleague told me about an unusual nutritionist who had helped her eat better and, in the process, she'd lost a lot of weight. I made an appointment immediately.

On my intake form I revealed that the last time I'd been to a doctor had been twenty years earlier. When Dr. Jairo Rodriguez raised his eyebrows I admitted that I really don't like (as in trust) doctors. Perhaps in an effort to relax me, he changed the subject and asked me how I was feeling.

"Exhausted," I answered, but quickly qualified that. "I have a small business. Don't you think most people who have small businesses in New York are totally exhausted all the time?"

He smiled and said, "Oh well, would you like a drink of water?"

"Um, sure."

As he handed me a glass of water he asked me to drink it slowly with my head tilted back. When I put the glass down he said, "Well, you're really not going to like doctors now because I have to tell you that you have a tumor on your thyroid gland."

Just like that I found out I literally had a lump in my throat, which was clearly visible, moving up and down, as I was swallowing the water. Dr. Rodriguez told me that we wouldn't know how serious it was (cancer versus no big deal) until the results of a thorough blood test came back. I started sweating and wondered how much blood is required for a thorough blood test.

After the needles went in and back out, I was invited into Dr. Rodriguez's office where he told me it might be possible to dissolve the lump in a natural way, through diet and supplements. He pulled out a folder and wrote my name on the top of it. He wanted me to start the extensive program of food and vitamin therapy that was outlined in detail in the folder.

He opened to the first page and I saw a long list of foods. He began personalizing it for me by crossing things off the list. "Dairy is out, beans are in, sugar is out—and that means no fruit, no carrots, no beets, or corn—meat is in, olives are out, salad dressing is out, and alcohol is out!"

His pen was zipping across that paper so fast I think I was in shock. Finally he flipped back to the cover and wrote at the top: "1,300 calories a day; lunch and dinner allow one serving of fish or chicken no bigger than the size of your palm." He looked up at me and, perhaps in response to the expression on my face, said sympathetically, "You may have one piece of bread at dinner and one portion of rice or potatoes the size of your fist."

He patted the cover of the folder with upbeat energy, ready to send me off on my new life. "Any questions?"

"Well, at least I'll lose some weight."

"Oh, you will!" He scribbled something on the booklet cover again and turned it toward me. TLG. "That's what you are going to be: Thin, Lean, and Gorgeous!"

Ewww. Talk about a mixed message. Two minutes ago Jairo is telling me that I need to change my diet in order to save my life and now it's all about skinny = gorgeous. Sigh. That thing again. I guess I set myself up for this by going to a doctor known for helping people lose weight. But this kind of approach was really not good for me, especially coming from a health professional. I needed encouragement to get healthy, not more reinforcement of my already troubled body image. Sure, I wanted to lose weight but I didn't know if I was up for going on a totally antisocial diet.

In the meantime, Dr. Rodriguez was still talking so fast that I regretted not bringing a notebook along as my friend had recommended, warning me I'd never catch all his analysis and instructions otherwise. I think Dr. Rodriguez could see that I was spinning because he shifted gears and slowed down his pace. He actually took a breath, looked at me, and in a soft, caring voice said, "You know, it isn't your fault."

To my surprise, I started to cry. How did he know I thought that?

"Your thyroid hasn't been working properly for a long time. Gaining weight is not your fault."

His words helped me realize how mean I had been to myself. Just like my mom hating herself for losing control of her body, I had also spent so much time blaming myself for something I couldn't control, not realizing that I'd been getting sick, too. These words from the doctor were an epiphany after all the frustration and confusion and blame I'd been loading onto myself for so many years.

Dr. Rodriguez understood this. He was intense but he was also kind, and his program gave me a clear path toward feeling in control of my body. He told me that depending on the seriousness of the official diagnosis, I might have to have surgery or take drugs for the rest of my life. I don't know if I could have stuck with such a restrictive diet plan or managed to down ten vitamins every morning, noon, and night just for vanity's sake, but highly motivated by fear of cancer, I signed on.

Part of the reason was I trusted Dr. Rodriguez. Not only was he kind and caring; he was handsome and fit and vibrant. That inspired me! Clearly he knew what he was talking about, even though it turned out that he was a chiropractor and not an M.D. He told me that his actual title was biochemical specifist, which means he was custom-making my special diet and supplement program based on my personal health scenario. After my blood tests came back, he would tweak it further, depending on what he learned.

Over the next five months, I lost nearly fifteen pounds, which isn't really that much considering I followed the diet precisely. I never cheated even though I got so hungry at first that I had a headache and felt really desperate. As instructed, I called Dr. Rodriguez after the first five days and when he asked if I had any questions, I had just one: Can I have a snack? I told him that when most people were sitting down to dinner at around six P.M., I was just walking into my studio to teach an evening yoga class on a very empty, hungry stomach. He allowed me to have a bagel or a yogurt. I didn't really understand why a bagel was okay, since he restricted both my sugar and carb intake, but I didn't want to ask him about it in case he changed his mind. Oh, but I did have one more question: How long would I have to keep up this diet? He lowered his voice like a Halloween spook and said, "Forever." Very funny, Dr. Rodriguez.

When my blood results came back, Dr. Rodriguez told me I had an autoimmune disease called Hashimoto's Thyroiditis and he sent me to a thyroid specialist who confirmed the diagnosis. Jairo warned me that I would probably need to begin taking daily medication, most likely for the rest of my life, and he was right about that, too. I began a daily regimen of taking synthetic thyroid medication but I also followed Jairo's recommendation that I stick with the diet.

And, surprisingly, I had gotten used to this diet. Even going to restaurants was no problem because I found it a fun challenge to see if I could create a "legal" meal from any menu. About two months after I started the Jairo diet, as David and I called it, we attended a fancy dinner and performance to benefit my Buddhist practice group. We sat at a table with the VP of Artists & Repertoire for a major record label; the producer for a famous classical composer; and a super-rich businessman focusing on green initiatives and his wife, who recently developed a health-care curriculum for trauma care workers. Everyone was a Buddhist and this was a high-end Buddhist schmoozatorium. There was nothing I could eat except half the breast of chicken and sparkling water. And I was fine with that. I didn't mind the antisocial aspect of not eating like a normal person. In fact, I felt righteous and clean.

But, in the end, that just became another kind of craving. Because righteous and clean is not a balanced way to be, any more than feeling guilty and dirty. It didn't allow for any slippage. There were no soft edges, no ease. It seems I felt safest when I was like Leroy: just doing—as in eating—exactly the same thing all the time. But life isn't like that. Everything in life ebbs and flows, including my body, and that is how it should be. Stability doesn't come from holding on to extremes. It comes from riding the waves, not holding the water. The very word *balance* comes from the Latin word *balare*, which means "to dance." After a while, I needed more movement.

Over time, I began to replace the skim in my morning coffee with half and half, I allowed myself a glass of wine once in a while, and sometimes I would share a dessert with a friend. None of this is all that bad, and if I could have just relaxed, it would have been fine.

But along with letting myself go back to some comfort food

now and then, something else came back, too—old feelings of shame. Whenever I veered from the diet rules, I got nervous. I would feel around for any new softness or bloating and the next morning that old recording would start to play, reviewing what I ate the night before and vowing to do better today. In a way, that is exactly what Mark Bittman is suggesting, only without the bad vibes attached. But since my addiction was to the drama of it all, it just flared right up again, like an addiction relapse.

Once I realized that I didn't have cancer and that my condition was manageable, my intention shifted from being healthy back to the more familiar, more materialistic goal of TLG. I played right into Jairo's trip, which played right into my addiction to wanting my body to be different.

At first, I experienced a certain sense of confidence just from feeling so thin and light, but over time this relationship inverted. The more weight I lost, the more fragile my confidence became, as if I were looking over my shoulder to see what might sabotage the whole thing. The great feeling of being a TLG goddess had been hard earned and I was paranoid that it would be taken from me at any time. I wasn't relaxed. I was vigilant. I didn't trust myself; I was afraid that I might lose my discipline, giving my power to the food instead of myself. This led me right back to an obsession, not with eating food but with thinking about food and constantly planning what I could eat when and how much. In the end, I felt the same way I'd felt before I lost the weight: totally preoccupied with my body. I might have felt a sense of detoxified cleanliness but it was tinged with the unclean feelings of shame that accompanied the tiniest cheat. Is it surprising that over time I gained back all that weight and more?

But I didn't see this happening at the time. As instructed, I continued reporting back to Jairo every five weeks. He would take me into a little examination room where I took off my shoes and stood on the big medical scale for my weigh-in. Then I took off my socks and lay down on a chiropractic table while Jairo unwrapped the cords of a small electronic measuring device that looked like an EKG machine. He attached plastic electrodes to my feet and hands and asked me the same question every time.

"What's your age?"

Every time I told him my age, he acted shocked, as if he had never known it before.

"You look fantastic! You're a gorgeous woman!"

He inputted my age and weight into the device, pushed some buttons, and a piece of paper rolled out of the machine, like a taxi receipt. I got up, put my socks on and went back into his office for the moment of truth. The printout revealed whether I had eaten sugar in the previous twenty-four hours and other details such as my current fat content. He was pleased with my results. My thyroid numbers were within the healthy range and I had achieved the state of TLG. I always left the office of Dr. Rodriguez feeling as fantastic as he told me I looked. I'm not sure if he was flirting with me but it felt like it, and each time he told me how good I looked, his words gave me validation. I always walked out the door onto Central Park West feeling sexy and powerful, for the moment.

In the end, though, I stopped seeing Jairo because I couldn't maintain the repressive nature of the diet, and I was gagging on all those vitamins I had to take daily. I did continue taking the one thyroid pill each morning, which perked up my metabolism. I'd told Dr. Rodriguez at my first appointment that I was exhausted and later I learned that it is not uncommon for people with this disease to be misdiagnosed as having chronic fatigue syndrome.

Although at first I was freaked out about having to take a pill every day for the rest of my life, I began to have more sustained energy and I wondered how I had managed to accomplish so much with an underactive thyroid. But it's not a magic pill. It doesn't make you thin. It just prevents Hashimoto's from leading to something worse, like heart failure.

My failure was of a different nature. I'd lost what my Buddhist teachers would call primordial confidence. Primordial confidence doesn't depend on us doing something worthy. This confidence is our birthright as humans; it is the confidence we deserve based on the fact that we are born and are good at our core. But my confidence was not primordial; it was conditional. And whether I was thin or not thin, whatever shape my body took, at my core I had no confidence. I didn't trust myself to take care of myself properly, and I felt good only when somebody else told me I looked good.

I had lost trust in my own Basic Goodness.

———— ✦ ————

One of the most important lessons in my teacher training program is called the 3Cs: confidence, clarity, and compassion. These are the qualities of a good yoga teacher and exactly what I am trying to exude as I lead my intermediate-level students into an arm balancing posture called Bakasana or Crow Pose. It's a new pose for them and I know from experience that if I demonstrate it first, some of them will just sit down in defeat without even trying. So I'm not going to demonstrate it at all. I'm going to sneak them into this pose.

This is where confidence, clarity, and compassion overlap. I have confidence that I can teach them how to do this pose or at least how to approach it. That confidence is built on the fact that I plan to take them along step-by-step with clear instructions and that I will let them know they can go just as far as they like and it's always fine to go no further. That's the compassion part.

The reason the 3Cs are so important for a yoga teacher is that these are the qualities I want to transmit to the students and Crow Pose is a good vehicle for this goal.

Thirty-five students are sitting on the floor with their legs extended straight out in front of them.

"Everyone, please bend your knees and lean back on your hands."

They can do this easily and, in fact, love doing it because it is a good core strengthener and even yogis like having firm abdominals.

"Lift your right foot off the floor, and then your left foot."

They follow along, so far so good.

"Now lift your arms up off the floor and extend them forward at shoulder height. From here bend your arms so your palms face forward and say, "Whoa"

"Whoa!" They all do it and start laughing, which makes some of the students tip over. No problem. They roll back up into position and join the other thirty people balancing on their sitting bones in a position very similar to my old John F. Kennedy President's Fitness Club exercise, also called the V-Sit.

"Okay, keep your feet together, flexed, as if you were standing on them. Now bring your right elbow to the inside of your right knee."

That elicits a few more uninvited whoas and even more when I ask them to do the same gesture with their left leg—at the same time! This is getting challenging but I know they love it and that this is actually part of the path toward developing the confidence they need to do the full Crow Pose.

"Good, everybody, yes! Keep your feet together . . . and exhale and release your legs back to the floor. Lean back on your elbows and shake your legs out for a moment."

Didn't have to ask twice. That was the compassion part, too.

"Now we will do this same pose only you will be standing on your hands instead of sitting on your feet."

I'm not surprised that some balk at this while others pop up onto their feet ready to give it a go. They try tucking their elbows inside their knees and standing on their hands but most of them can't get airborne.

"My abs are too weak."

"My hips are too tight."

"My arms aren't strong enough."

Experience has told me these comments would come up.

"It doesn't really matter if your arms are weak or your abs are weak or your hips are tight. This pose, like every pose in yoga, is about how all things are working together. Have you ever noticed a person who has a great vibe, exudes friendliness and confidence, someone you feel magnetized toward? And then on second glance, if you felt like being hyper-critical and not so nice, you might notice that their chin is too small or their nose is too big or something like that? In other words, this pose is greater than the sum of its parts!

"In fact, you could even say that none of these obstacles exist because Crow Pose is about how all of these parts—arms, hips, abs, and legs and breath and concentration—come together for that moment, and that's what makes it yoga."

I ask them to come into a low squat on a yoga block and curl their back, making their body into a little round ball shape.

"Lean forward and place your hands on the floor."

They can do this.

"Scooch your shoulders inside your thighs."

They can also do this.

"Slowly, super slowly, begin to shift your weight onto your hands. Just a little bit. Now lift your right foot up off the block. Replace it to the block. Lift your left foot off the block for a breath . . . and replace it to the block. Relax."

They step off their blocks feeling the beginning of satisfaction mixed with enthusiasm. They are almost doing the full Crow Pose but they still haven't gotten both feet in the air at the same time.

"So how was that?" I want to check in with them before taking them to the next step.

"I'm scared of falling on my head."

"Me, too!"

Lots of nodding heads.

"Yes, I don't blame you. This is a pretty out-of-the-box thing to be doing and to tell you the truth, you might fall on your head. I fell on my head several times when I was learning this pose. But I have a tip for you. Fold up two blankets and put them on the floor in front of you, like this."

I pull over two folded Mexican yoga blankets and squat down into a little ball. Then I shift my weight forward and lift one foot, then the other. I join my flexed feet together as if I were standing on them and say, "And then if you do fall over, this will happen." And I lean forward so far that the top of my head goes boop, right down onto the blanket.

Everyone cracks up because the fall is so anticlimactic. I pop up with a big smile.

"Wanna try it?"

And they do and some get up and some don't get up but I see their confidence showing. I think to myself, "They really were listening when I told them that practice is about expanding your comfort zone." I watch them going slowly, working with clarity and curiosity about how to fulfill each step along the way, instead of trying to skip ahead to the end goal. I am happy to see them being generous with themselves, compassionate about what they are able to do today.

———— ◆ ————

My friend Jamie has tons of confidence. She's been in the public eye most of her life and has learned how to balance positive attention and notoriety. At fifty-two, she knows who her friends are and where her priorities lie. I know that she's worked hard to create these healthy equations in her life, so I went to California to get her advice on the subjects of body image, self-confidence, and goodness.

Her sexy body is only one of the reasons Jamie Lee Curtis is famous. She is also known for her comedic talent; her graceful transition to middle age; and her relevant, inspirational children's books. Among her friends she is famous for being generous, honest, and supremely organized.

These last three qualities were on full display the day I went to her house to talk with her about being a woman—a famous woman—in a body. We've been friends for nearly two decades, piggybacking on the lifelong relationship between our husbands. Not only had Jamie instantly agreed to talk with me about her relationship with her body, but she turned it into a special evening by inviting David and me to come by for another thing she is famous for among her friends, a healthy and delicious home-cooked meal.

Our flight from NYC was four hours late so instead of a refreshing few hours at the hotel, we shuttled to the rental car and called Jamie, who guided us along back streets to avoid the worst of the LA rush hour traffic. Although I felt crumpled and a tad travel worn, the fresh air coming off the ocean and the mellow early evening light was revitalizing. I rolled the windows down and got high on the SoCal ambience. There were the Pep Boys: Manny, Moe, and Jack; the friendly Giant Donut still sitting atop that tiny donut shop since the seventies; esoteric religions cheek-to-jowl with manicure salons; and bumper-to-bumper traffic with no pedestrians to be seen anywhere. We turned the corner past Bikram's Yoga College of India and I wondered if Jamie was still taking yoga classes there.

We finally rolled down the driveway into a quiet, flowering backyard and as we walked up the steps into the heart of the house, the kitchen, Jamie greeted us with hugs and kisses. The four of us hung out in her spacious, hyper-functional, spic-and-span kitchen for a while having sparkling water, homemade hummus, and warm pita triangles. Then my husband pulled out his guitar, her husband pulled out his mandolin, and Jamie and I walked into her office as they started picking bluegrass in the background.

In the years that I've known Jamie, her body, like mine and those of all my women friends, has waxed and waned. She's been on a diet now and then, got sober about ten years ago, sometimes does yoga—the same things that many of my friends have gone through but with one major difference. She's done it all publicly.

I knew that Jamie wouldn't hold anything back and so I started right out by mentioning "True Thighs," the 2002 *More* magazine piece in which she modeled her "real" body. She would get there eventually but I guess I shouldn't have been surprised that when the subject of body image came up, her first topic was her mother [Janet Leigh], who had very recently passed away.

"I just wrote a magazine article about my mother; about my mother's body and her relationship with her body. I actually used the words 'the most intimate relationship my mother had was with her own body.' Then I changed it because I worried that it would become a pull quote. I didn't want those words to become the cause célèbre of a loving memory of my mother. Yet it was intimate, her relationship with her body.

"When a woman's commodity is her body . . . and she gains her fame from her body . . . such as athletes do—"

I chimed in, "Like me. I was a dancer and now I'm a yoga teacher."

She nods but doesn't stop. She's on a roll with a subject that she has thought about a lot. "Their bodies—I don't want to say betrayed them because they weren't betrayed—their bodies changed as bodies change. But their mental relationship with the body is complicated, more complicated than necessarily for a normal woman who has had a couple of kids, went through the normal post-baby weight gain and attempted loss, and woke up middle-aged."

Now it was me nodding. "Sure, I get it. The pressure is less intense for an 'average' woman because her body is not going to be the cause of her losing her job or having people write about her."

Jamie tucks one leg under her and leans back to consider. "It's the mental attachment to it. I saw it happening a long time ago. I wrote a poem when I was twenty called 'I Felt My Body Go Today.'"

I felt my body go today,
or was it yesterday,
I don't know
I just know it's not the same,
you see it now in younger years,
they say it's in the air,
I say it's up here,
Your brain is where decay begins . . .

She peters out for a minute, trying to remember the rest of a poem she wrote thirty years earlier. And I'm as amazed that she picked this poem out of her memory as the fact that she was dealing with this issue at the age of twenty.

She gets the gist of it back. "And there was something about when old people show a picture to a young person and you're looking at a paper bag who says that was me, and you go, yeah right—in your dreams.

"So I was aware of this from a young age when I was just

starting to be known for my figure. It wasn't for my great beauty; it was for my figure.

"There was *Trading Places, Perfect,* and *True Lies*—that trip-tych of film work sort of solidified my cinema body as being amazing, and believe me, if I watch *Perfect* today"—here she pauses for dramatic effect—"I sit there saying, 'Unbelievable. That's unbelievable . . .' I would hate me! I would be saying, 'I hate you!'"

We're both laughing now because it's funny and also it feels good to be so honest. It feels good to admit that we're jealous of younger perfect bodies—even if one of those bodies was one of us!

Jamie can laugh at herself because she also remembers what it took to be so perfect. "I remember watching aerobics teach-ers who used to wear three pairs of those Lycra tights. It was the beginning of Lycra. I remember in the changing room seeing these women pulling on three pairs of Lycra tights to get that firm, smooth appearance. And I remember that even then Lycra was a tool to disguise.

"I remember going to Bikram's yoga class. He didn't let you wear anything on your legs. I wore tights and he said, 'Take them off' and I said, 'Excuse me?' and he repeated, 'No tights.'"

"How old were you then?"

"In my early twenties. In a leotard with no tights on. I thought, 'Oh my God.' Even then in my twenties, I was like ewaahhh!"

"So, did you do it?"

"Oh, sure, you had to. And you know what? Somebody actually wrote anonymously in one of these Beverly Hills newspapers—I think it was the *Beverly Hills Courier*—'There's a young movie actress who's supposed to be "perfect" and I saw her in a leotard and she certainly wasn't.'

"It was so snarky. I pretended I didn't even see the item, but afterward being outside in bare legs was not something that ever felt comfortable."

As she got up to check on the progress of dinner, she turned back for one last word. "Ever."

Jamie was preparing salmon to be cooked on cedar planks along with a veggie salad from a Jamie Oliver cookbook. As always her energy was high, her concentration was clear, and she was efficient at multitasking.

She looked better than ever, dressed in a navy blue shirt with the sleeves rolled up to three-quarter length and matching capris. She looked relaxed with a light, springtime-fresh manicure and pedicure, and I thought, "Actually, the way she looks *right now* is perfect."

I guess I shouldn't have been surprised to learn that just because she got such positive attention for her beautiful body, Jamie didn't ever feel completely comfortable exposing it. People think the same thing about me. I'm a yoga teacher, for goodness' sakes! I can stand on my head, hands, forearms, and shoulders for as long as I want and all the while appear to be calm and centered. No one can tell that when I'm doing a deep side bend I'm obsessing on that little flesh blob between my ribs and my hips. I don't think about the sleek feeling of the other side of my body, the side that is getting stretched and lengthened. No, I always tend to focus on the squish, the "imperfection." So why would it be any different for a movie star?

She came back with refills of sparkling water and I wondered out loud whether her physical discomfort led her to work extra hard on getting that perfect body. I wanted to know how she balanced the feeling of self-consciousness with being able to accept a starring role in a movie called *Perfect*.

"I didn't work hard. I did a minimum amount. I was never an athlete. I never ran. I never got on a treadmill. I never broke a sweat. The only sweat I used to break was in an aerobics class where you jump around and you get your heart rate going and your hair gets wet and you feel good."

"Feeling good is one thing, but did you also know you looked good?"

"Yeah, I knew that . . ."

"So you did have a certain level of confidence . . . ?"

"I was not particularly comfortable in my own skin, but I could manage it. My metabolism was great. I have a lot of energy. I have more energy than any human being I've ever met. My metabolism is just burning it. I never have to worry about it. But when I made *Perfect*, I knew that if I ate too much I'd get a little poochy tummy. I knew it. So I sort of didn't eat much. I mean, I was controlling what I ate even then and I was twenty-five years old."

By her thirties, she was a mom, having first adopted Annie in 1986 and adopting Tom ten years later. Though she continued appearing in films—often, by her account, "wearing support panty hose"—as her focus shifted away from her own physical upkeep, she found she didn't have the time or the inclination to exercise regularly.

"Support panty hose?" I made a face.

"Now people want to be in soft cotton clothes. But every foundation garment—like women wore back in the day—squeezes you. If you understand anything about physics, when you squeeze, something else expands. So many young girls are in these super-tight tank tops, but even those girls, if they're wearing a bra, they have a little back fat because their clothes are too tight."

I know exactly what she's talking about, so I jump in.

"It seems to me that some women don't care. They don't care if their back fat shows or their muffin tops show. I guess they either think that's sexy or that it's just normal or they say sure there's a little 'pineapple' there because that's your bra, like it's no big deal. But I always had this feeling that I would die of humiliation if I had back fat. Maybe they don't have as much body awareness or they weren't an actor or a dancer or—"

She sits up and interrupts. "Or"—important pause for effect—"maybe they feel so loved. And their husband thinks that they are the most beautiful woman that man has ever seen."

Another pause. Of course, she's right. Doesn't that seem simple enough? If someone tells you that you are beautiful and very obviously loves you exactly as you are, why would you obsess about a tiny bit of soft flesh? As if that were the one detail that would make someone love you or not love you. I guess I hadn't yet figured out that until we love ourselves, we can't experience or accept the love of others. Until then, we can't relax, even about a tiny bit of soft flesh here or there. We must be vigilant because there is a strong—even if it's unarticulated—delusion that only when our body is perfect in every way can we be loved.

I asked her, "But why is that not always enough for everyone? I know that one of the things that creates suffering is when people put all their happiness eggs in one basket—when I have a baby, when I get a dog, when I get this job, when I have the perfect body, then I will be happy. It just puts all that pressure on that one thing, and nothing can fulfill it, especially no relationship. You wouldn't expect that of your husband."

Jamie was reminded of a particularly dark episode. "I was going to go do a movie where I had to wear a bathing suit and instead of just committing to three months with a trainer and saying to myself, 'Cut out this, this, and this and you can drop twenty pounds. You can firm it all up, you know. You've got very good form under there.' Instead, I went to plastic surgery, because it was the easy, quick fix . . . And, it didn't work.

"That was really the beginning of a downward spiral that ended after I got sober. It ended about ten years ago and it ended because I went to Greece."

Great segue. She can really tell a story. Greece had come up earlier because that's where she learned to make that delicious hummus, which reminded her to pop back into the kitchen and check on the dinner. Then, she's back.

"On my trip to Greece with my sister and friends," she reminds me, "I was so uncomfortable in my body. It was the beginning of paparazzi, and it was just when it was really getting kind of bad. I went to the surf shop and bought these full-length pants that could get wet. I wore them to beaches because I didn't want anybody to take my picture in a bathing suit.

"But when I got back from that trip I was humiliated by my attempts to hide my body, and I was only forty years old."

That was how *More* came to publish what might be the most

famous article in the history of the magazine. "Jamie Lee Curtis wants to expose herself to you," the piece, titled "True Thighs," begins. "It is, she says, the only way to make things right."

And that's exactly what happened. "We knew the article was important," Susan Crandell, then editor-in-chief of *More*, told the *San Francisco Chronicle*. "But we didn't know how huge it would be. Even a twenty-three-year-old assistant at the *Today* show, after we were on last week, said the article made her feel so much better about her body."

Indeed, Jamie intended her bold statement to inspire. "I did the *More* photo session because I was promoting and talking about my fifth book, *I'm Gonna Like Me*, which was about self-esteem. I felt like it would be a real mistake to talk to children about self-esteem and not acknowledge that I had some issues of my own."

I prompted her to continue. "So, even after the enthusiastic reception, you still felt like a fraud?"

She gave me a you-got-it look. "I'm writing about self-esteem and advocating that you like yourself and love yourself and are self-accepting. And, here I am . . ." She pauses.

I finish her sentence for her. ". . . wearing pants to the beach."

"Right after the *More* piece came out, a tabloid published a picture of me from Greece, climbing out of the water at a pier, at a small little town in the middle of nowhere where we went to the water's edge. I love to dive into the water, and I dove into the water and swam around in my pants. And as I was climbing out I was reaching up to somebody to pull me up and somebody took a picture of me and the tabloid wrote, 'Weight a Minute, Is That Who I Think It Is?'"

As she scrolls her computer mouse to pull up the picture

from her super-organized photo archives, she says, "It was a very unflattering photograph. I look as big as a house. It's a bad angle and I'm soaking wet." The photo comes up and I see what she means.

We sit looking at each other for a moment. What a drag that must have been! We've all had bad photos taken and in these days of Facebook, I know I've had way too many unattractive photos posted of me and I hate it. But still, not that many people really look at pictures of me. I could only imagine the level of unwanted attention that photo must have brought to Jamie. But just as I'm thinking this, she sits forward a little because now she wants to deliver the clincher, the punch line of the story.

"Had that photograph appeared and had I *not* made this commitment to kind of out myself for it, I think I would have been devastated. I think I would have felt such shame. Instead, I was like, 'Fuck you!' I already did it. I already got it. I already got this handled, thank you very much.

"And then the *More* thing was insane. I didn't expect that. I didn't go into that thinking, 'This is going to be a big deal.' I knew women would relate. I knew women would appreciate it. It's like doing a kindness for something and saying, 'Oh, by the way, in case you've ever looked at me and gone, like, whoa . . .'"

Yeah, I got it and I'm on board. "Don't bother hating me because . . ."

"Yeah, don't be a hater because I got it, too." She sits back. She's not smug at all, just feeling good about having delivered her message.

I loved the whole thing. She figured out how to encourage and help others and, at the same time, to grow her own power.

Always one to acknowledge bodhisattvic activity, I complimented her. "Jamie, it was perfect because it was doing a good
deed for everyone including yourself."

She doesn't want to go there. "But there *was* fraud with it,
too. The fraud was, I was saying, 'This is what I look like.' I'm
this age. I've got two kids. I have a marriage. I work at my kids'
school. I don't have the time to do things like some of these
actresses who blog and write about their workout regimes and
their private yoga teachers and their colonics and their this and
their that. I don't have that because I'm like you. I'm a mom. I'm
working and so 'I'm unwilling'"—and then she pauses to
emphasize—"not 'I can't,' but 'I'm unwilling to give the amount
of time necessary to perfect my body. So this is what I look like.
Here it is right there.'

"But what happened was women started coming up to me
and saying, 'High five, be the way we are!! Love you, honey.
You're real! Your shape doesn't matter.'"

Now I was the one sitting forward in my seat. Why did that
kind of feedback make her feel less authentic?

She continued, "Then, two things happened. One, another
tabloid picture appeared that said, 'Weight Watchers.' They put
a number next to my picture that said that I weighed a hundred
sixty-one pounds."

I felt outraged for her. "How can they know how much you
weigh?"

"I went home, got on the scale. One hundred sixty-one
pounds! And I thought, Oh my goodness me. This is what happens when you say"—she makes a kissing sound—"'I am what I
am. I eat what I eat. I eat what I want. I eat granola and Wheat

Thins. That's good for you and this is the way I am.' And then"—
she slows down the rant and gets reflective about how she hadn't
really taken care of herself during that five-year period—"I
thought, I'm forty-five years old. What am I going to weigh at
fifty-five? Am I going to weigh one-seventy, one-eighty? Am I
going to get into my seventies and weigh even more?"

Her energy levels, she went on to confess, had flagged. She
didn't want to exercise. "My cholesterol level was ridiculous,
and I was unhealthy."

She decided to get healthy. Taking the approach of caring
for herself, which included losing a little weight, began a real
shift for Jamie. She realized that the amount of bread and flour
and rice and pasta that she had been eating was not good for
her, especially since without exercising it just turned into sugar
and was making her overweight. She started eating a more
protein-heavy diet, and slowly began to cut out what was bad
for her. She did it in a reasonable time frame so that she didn't
feel deprived. She incorporated exercise.

"I have a layer of fat that will never go away. I also have
completely understood that I am a Hungarian Jew from Buda-
pest. I go to the gym now three times a week and"—she ges-
tures to her triceps flap—"this will never go away. I don't care if
I lost thirty pounds; this will never go away. I rarely wear a tank
top because I just don't think it looks particularly attractive on
me. But I don't feel like I'm hiding anything. I feel like I look
good. I feel good. I'm not obsessed about it. I get on the scale
and I have a five-pound window."

A five-pound window! She figured out what Collette—the
silver-haired woman in the pedicure salon who'd told me she

thought of women's bodies like waxing and waning moons—had figured out; that five pounds this way and that is not drama worthy. It's normal. Instead of freaking out when the scale moves around inside that window, why not build that into your list of appropriate body options?

I wanted to compliment Jamie again, to reiterate how great I thought it was that she's learned to take care of herself so well, but the time for talking about it all seemed to have passed. Jamie's attention was on her computer. She clicks to bring up another photo, this one of her diving off the pier into the water, instead of climbing out. She's wearing a real bathing-suit bottom that beautifully highlights her sleek, well-defined hips and legs. In this picture, she looks graceful and elegant, flying through the air like a dolphin. She wraps up our chat with a happy ending. "Now I am much more comfortable in my own skin at fifty-two."

And with that, we called the husbands and sat down to dinner. The conversation went in completely different directions at that point, but I was quiet most of the evening. As I ate the light summery dessert—a thin shortcake biscuit with raspberries and two drips of cream—I felt full of respect and admiration for my friend who had learned how to occupy her own body and maintain her confidence, whether nice or not-so-nice things were being said about her body.

———•✦•———

Lola, Tia, Jules, and I gathered together around an earthy wooden table above the beach on the Nosara Peninsula of Costa Rica. We see one another for a week each year, as part of the annual Omega winter retreat. As our men gathered across the terrace, we sat down together, letting the warm winter night air thaw our cold Northeast bones.

One of the best things about our friendship is that since we don't see one another very often, we don't do small talk. We talk about what we've been learning and practicing; what we've discovered or created; and what we've been able to let go of. As part of my quest for advice from other women, I asked them how they felt about their bodies.

A silence opened up and we sat together comfortably, feeling okay with the spaciousness. Lola is a big blonde who didn't seem to mind wearing a bikini when we went sailing last year, even though I knew from her husband that she was unhappy with her weight; Jules is a petite woman who got breast implants as a gift for her now ex-boyfriend; and Tia, the most voluptuous of us all, is a real dakini, with long hair and a zaftig body, always in red, black, or white flowing skirts and lacy tunics. These were my three annual female friends: a store owner; a massage therapist; an author. And then there's me—the yoga teacher who hates her body, never wants to be seen in a bathing suit, and always wears baggy yoga clothes.

Lola answered my question by telling us a story about a woman who came into her shop in Rhinebeck. The woman tried on a dress and then stood right out in the middle of the store, admiring herself in the mirror. She ran her hands up and down her body and purred, saying, "Wow. I look so good in this dress."

"And she really did look good! Everyone in the shop was looking at her and loving her attitude."

I chimed in: "That's cool. I mean, it's practically illegal in our society to actually say right out loud that you think you look good."

That's when Lola delivered the kicker. "Yeah, and she was seventy years old!"

Oh, somehow that detail changed the whole story. I wondered out loud, "Do you think you would have had the same response to a twenty-five- or thirty-five- or forty-five-year-old woman who publicly admired herself?"

Lola thought about it for a moment and said, "I would still think 'good for you!'"

I dared to be totally honest by saying, "Well, it's not something I like to admit, but maybe at the same time I would be thinking, 'I don't like women like that.' Right? I don't know why women compare themselves to each other, instead of just having our own confidence."

Perhaps I was just ranting on about my own internal drama, but everybody knew what I was talking about. Then Lola offered up another story. She told us we should make a point of going to this little dress shop in Nosara. "You have to meet this clothing designer. She is really good at helping you find things that look amazing on your body, usually things you wouldn't normally even think of trying on." Lola told us how the designer talked her into trying on a beautiful dress, although it was sleeveless, backless, and very cleavage-y—three things she never wears. To her surprise, she loved how the dress looked on her and she took the leap and bought it.

That night she went to a party and there was another woman in a red version of the same dress. Lola didn't mind that there was another person in the same dress, but she didn't like the way the dress looked on that other woman. And then suddenly she was sure she also must not look good in that dress. Her confidence tanked as she realized she was at a party in a sleeveless, backless, low-cut dress that was all wrong for her. She caved in her chest, hugged her shawl around her shoulders and decided she would never wear that dress again.

Yeah. Got it. We all got that whole story. We knew exactly how Lola felt. Why is our confidence so fragile?

I asked them, "Can you imagine what it would feel like to have the body confidence of the woman in Lola's shop?"

As a rebuttal to the confidence comment, Jules said, "I think I look good for my age."

Openhearted Lola said she thought we all looked pretty good for our ages and that, in fact, we were all exceptionally young looking.

"I agree," I said, wanting to show that I can be positive and supportive to my women friends, "but what would it take for us to say we look good—period. Without that 'for my age' part?"

"Hmmmmm . . ." Jules squirmed a little bit.

I asked them to visualize themselves being happy in their bodies and what that would look like.

"What about you, Tia?"

I was so curious to hear what she would say. Tia has a completely adoring husband and sometimes after dinner she puts on her ankle bells and entertains us with ultra-womanly Indian Kathak dancing. When she's not writing books and giving workshops, she designs her own white, red, or black lace tunics and takes care of her ponies.

She smiled. "I guess I should probably think about my body

more. I don't know. . . . But when I visualize being happy what comes to mind is lightness."

What did she mean by that? To feel light. When I looked at Tia she didn't look heavy or light. She is not thin. But I don't think that is what she meant. I've thought about this so many times since that night and now I think I understand.

I don't think Tia meant light, as in poundage, but rather energetically light. Light in spirit. Not bogged down by things that don't matter. And you know, that really is how I think of Tia. Instead of focusing on her body, like the serious meditator she is, she consciously places her attention on what is happening in the moment—dancing, creativity, family, being helpful to others. I felt inspired by her comment and secretly thought, "I'll have what she's having."

But the part where she doesn't really think about her body? It reminded me of the Buddha and his early cohorts who said, "Let's deny the existence of our body because that is the source of our desire, and desire is the source of unhappiness." Is there a way to feel a lightness of being that acknowledges the body, that delights in the body, but does not limit that delight by applying it only to one size and shape of body?

When I got back to NYC I decided that, in a similar way of doing a thirty-day yoga challenge, I would do a thirty-day positive visualization challenge. I would consciously visualize my body as I want it to be for thirty days and see if it worked. But then I got stuck. Because what do I want it to look like? I don't know. I do know that I want to break out of the dead-end materialistic approach to life that feeds cravings, such as wanting to be more thin and more perfect. Wasn't I going for lightness from the inside out? What does that look like? So, if I let go of my habitual picture of the "perfect" body as my goal, then what picture should I paint instead?

I thought of a healthy body and I realized that I have that. I thought of a strong body and I have that, too. I thought of a younger body and knew I didn't want to go there. It was good to discover that I might envy younger women in a certain way, but I don't have an urge to torture myself about being the age that I am. I have gray hair now, which I am loving. So if I am strong, healthy, and okay with my age, then why am I not happy about my body? Like Tia, I want to feel and be light from the inside out. Does that mean I need to change my body or my mind, or both? If the body is heavy, can the mind be light? If the mind is heavy, can the body be light?

This thirty-day positive body visualization challenge felt like a koan; one of those mysterious Zen questions that doesn't have a straight answer. Instead of wondering about the sound of one hand clapping, I pondered:

What is the weight of one body of light?

or

If a body changes but no one notices, can it still become light?

Maybe, if the thirty-day challenge to visualize what my body would look like if I felt light is like a Zen puzzle, then I should try solving it like a Zen practitioner. That meant meditating.

———•◆•———

When I first sat sessin, an intense meditation retreat, at Dai Bosatsu Zendo, I was amazed to discover what a total baby I was. By that point, I'd been meditating for several years, practicing the mindfulness technique known as shamatha or calm abiding. In Zen this kind of sitting meditation is called zazen, and the actual meditation technique is nearly identical.

As my friend Enkyo Pat O'Hara Roshi says, "Begin with that part of your mind that you call your body." That means you begin by taking a good upright cross-legged position on the cushion. Turn your palms up and place one on top of the other. Keep your eyes halfway open and allow your gaze to rest on the floor. Consciously place your attention on your natural breath, feeling the sensation of the air going in and going out. The breath is used as a home base for the wandering mind because breathing can only happen now, never in the past or the future. Whenever you realize that your mind has strayed, you acknowledge that activity by saying to yourself, "Thinking," in a gentle, neutral inner voice. Then you return your attention to the sensation of the breath. That's it.

It's so simple that it's difficult. We all want to do it perfectly and tend to interpret it as having no thoughts. But mindfulness meditation is not about that at all. It is a practice for noticing when our mind gets caught up in thinking, which *is* about being in the past or future—regretting and reliving, or planning and rehearsing. This is a way to relax that habitual activity and return to the present, again and again. It's not about getting rid of thoughts, but about learning to work with the thoughts that we have naturally. The first step in doing that is to recognize when we have thoughts and how they pull us around. This simple technique involves noticing, letting go, and coming back—resisting attachment to any thought, whether positive or negative.

In this way, we begin to create a gap between a stimulus, like a thought, and its response, like saying something or doing something. Of course, we do need to think thoughts in order to function, but mostly our thoughts are habitual and are followed by speedy reactionary impulses. That is how those ruts we are stuck in get so deep.

We go through life bouncing around from one habitual reaction to the next and wonder why we feel powerless, unstable, and confused. Meditation practice is said to develop mental habits of strength, stability, and clarity, which are useful in off-the-cushion situations.

Even though my training up until this point had been in the Tibetan Buddhist lineage, I'd been invited to teach yoga as part of the zendo's late autumn sessin. I was warmly welcomed, shown to my room, and then the next thing I knew a robe was thrown over my shoulders and I was sitting in Sukhasana in the meditation hall. This strict Zen retreat allowed no talking and no moving. Tradition dictated that there was also no electricity so as the sun went down, the room got dark and the cold set in. I was lucky that my cushion faced the window because it was beautiful to see the snow falling outside, but I wished I was wearing long johns under my cotton robe. The Tibetan Buddhist middle-path approach allows for some physical shifting and I almost got up to get a sweater, but then I remembered where I was and stayed put.

I sat perfectly still. Up popped the thought, "I'm freezing!"

I came back to my breath. After hours of this, my commitment started to fade along with the winter light. I didn't always want to come back to the breath. I preferred to indulge in internal whining. No one can tell what you are thinking anyway, right? I let my mind go. "Why didn't they tell me there was no heat on this retreat? This isn't Japan in medieval times. Please. I hate this. I'm probably going to get a cold now. This is a drag. I can't believe this is just the first day." Eventually those thoughts just played themselves out, and I came back to the breath.

Other times, when I had more energy, more courage, more curiosity, I thought, "Wow, what a baby I am. I'm used to having my every sensation satisfied. I'm cold. Then, I'm hungry. Then, I'm tired. How interesting!" Then, I labeled all that thinking and came back to my breath. I started to become fascinated with how these habitual urges arose and then amazingly, if I didn't respond to them in any way, they passed on their own. Some took longer than others and it got increasingly more challenging to stay awake in the fading afternoon light after days of 4:20 A.M. wake-up gongs. But it was clear that feelings— emotional and physical—only do one thing and that is change. No need to get your knickers in a knot over an itch that is going to manage to scratch itself eventually.

In this way I started to gain confidence. I discovered that I didn't have to be a slave to my thoughts. I didn't even have to pay attention to them. All I had to do was stay steady.

On the middle evening of the retreat, the abbot of the temple, Eido Roshi, slowly walked through the meditation hall, followed by a monk who carried a paper lantern high on a stick. In his elegant, samurai-like brocades, Roshi passed by every meditator in the hall, making his rounds like a general inspecting the troops. As he passed me I felt moved by his grace and dignity. Nearly seventy years old, Roshi had been sitting this retreat along with us. Taking his place at the front, he let some moments of silence pass and then he gave us a Zen version of a pep talk. He acknowledged that deep practice was challenging but that many before us had done this thing, too. By fulfilling our commitment to create a quiet space and abiding in it together, we were developing spiritual maturity.

As a special treat, we were invited to hold out our empty cups. A senior monk spooned green powder into each cup held by two grateful hands over two crossed legs with aching knees, one after the next, down the row of cushions. Another monk passed along the line pouring hot water into each cup and a third monk whisked the green powder in every cup into a frothy green tea. We were offered one small chocolate each. Applying our mindfulness, we tasted our treats slowly and relished the intense richness of the green tea and chocolate. I felt content in this cold and dark, quiet, safe space.

As he got up to leave the meditation hall, Roshi's kindness came through beneath his dharma warrior toughness, honed from decades of practice in the fierce Rinzai Zen tradition. In a typical Japanese movie actor growl, he delivered one final encouragement, "Do your best!"

While I might not have been able to figure out what body I was going for in my thirty-day positive visualization challenge, I decided that what I could do was begin applying the mindfulness meditation technique to my grumpy inner voice—the one that had somehow come along in my luggage all the way to

Hong Kong and India. Why not use this method of labeling as an antidote to the unkind thoughts that arise about my body?

The more I thought about it, the more I was convinced that letting go of those thoughts was the only way to quiet the voice of my inner grump. I pledged to use my meditation practice to reduce the power of that worn-out thought path.

My thirty-day challenge would consist of allowing the sweat of my commitment to muddy those overused tracks, lessening their support for wrong thinking. If I could let the grass grow over those neuro-channels of judgment, eventually there would no longer be a clear way to cross that ground. Then, I could create a different map with a tender new trail, one that might not have a clear destination, but that held the promise of spacious, open-minded, non-judgmental positivity.

Isn't this why I'm practicing? Sitting on a cushion watching my breath for hours and days on end isn't so I can be the best meditator. It's practice for applying mindfulness to things that matter, to my real-life issues. I know in my gut this direction will lead to lightness and freedom. This time-tested method, passed down to me by Roshi and Rimpoche and all my precious teachers, will help lick my habit of hard thoughts. It's going to take time, but I'll be patient, remembering Roshi's advice. All I can do is my best.

———— •◆• ————

After the first five-minute session of sitting meditation, Bob, one of the students in the Yoga Body, Buddha Mind workshop, raised his hand. "I'm no good at this. I can't do it."

The notion of having to practice in order to sit still seems alien. Don't we all know how to sit still? Isn't that what we do when we are watching TV or doing our email? "If you're not good at this, what are you good at, Bob? What is it that you've mastered in your life?"

Bob sort of stared at me and everybody laughed, in a good-natured way, happy that they weren't being put on the spot. But I liked this idea. "Let's have every person here tell us what they have mastered!" I was excited!

At first, no one wanted to say anything. It's hard to admit that we are great at something. So I started it off by telling the class that I have mastered lying on the couch with a murder mystery, a cappuccino, and Leroy. If necessary, I can do it for hours!

Turns out the class included a master sleeper who can sleep so much that she even takes a three-hour pre-sleep nap before she goes to bed at night. There was a fire juggler—I noticed she was missing a large patch of hair on her head. There was a great mom, a great doggie dad, an expert in giving flu shots, and a person who always finds the perfect-sized plastic container for leftovers. One guy said he had mastered the art of living a balanced life.

How did we all get so good at these things? Repetition. Just from the doing. It's like yoga. In every class, day in and day out, I do the Sun Salutations. Over the years I've gained confidence in my ability to balance in off-balanced positions. I know I won't run out of breath or fall over, and even if I do, it doesn't matter. In fact that attitude is actually what makes me masterful in this arena.

As the students continued taking turns realizing and confessing their master crafts, my thoughts turned inward. I was not going to share this with my class, but I realized that repetition is how I've become such a masterful critic of every nook and cranny of my one precious body. Like any other skill set, if you practice it, you will improve it.

Science calls this ability neuroplasticity. That means that if we repeat a certain thought enough times, it creates a neural pathway. As we continue that thought pattern, the pathway gets stronger. The plasticity part is the good news: Because the brain is flexible—we can also change those pathways. If we shift our mind habits, we can create suppleness in the neural pathways and even create new ones that are more supportive of the way we want to be in the world. But like laying down a new road, it's not so easy to do, and pulling out the old well-worn track is even harder. It takes commitment and, yes, practice.

Everyone felt elated that they had outed their own masterfulness, and there was a genuine sense of rejoicing for one another's creativity and excellence.

"Okay, everyone. Let's try sitting still again for just five more minutes. Place your attention on your breath. When you realize you are thinking, gently let go of the thought and return your attention to your breath. With practice, you can do this, too."

———— • ✦ • ————

Millie had taken a turn for the worse. Following another fall, her body went into renal failure and her mind went who knows where. The doctors told me she was definitely going to pass away in the next three days and that I should make arrangements. With quivering hands and tears in my throat, I called the minister and the funeral home and her sister, Aunt Betty. But then Millie stabilized. She didn't pass away, but she hadn't come back to the world yet, either. I sat with her every day. It turns out that hospital rooms can be a good place to meditate, although sometimes I had to take a break. One day I stepped into the elevator and there was a friend.

Running into Nancy was like getting an IV of prana, a straight-up shot of life force. We were both running errands for our moms, mine in a bed on the geriatric ward and hers in the VIP suite, four floors above. Really, we were escaping the disease-laden corridors of New York Presbyterian Hospital into New York City's July heat wave. Normally oppressive in its thick stinkiness, on this day the slap of urban hotness felt good. Or at least it felt like something. Being in a hospital for a long time is like being in a bardo, the in-between place we hover in after death and before our next rebirth. Being outside and seeing Nancy reminded me that I was still alive, right here and now.

Theoretically a hospital is also a place of healing, and my mother was making minuscule improvement. But it is also a place that kills you after a while. Two weeks in the joint, and Millie had developed a patch of pneumonia on her lungs that Dr. Gopal, the beautiful dakini-faced child doctor, said she probably got from being in the hospital. I couldn't take my mom home yet, but I had to get out of there and so did Nancy.

After comparing notes on our respective mothers' progress, we went our separate ways—me to the bookstore and a cappuccino, Nancy off to the drugstore. But we ran into each other again on the way back into that white, noisy place, both pulling out our photo IDs as we walked past the security guards. She'd bought two tubes of arnica cream at the pharmacy, good for reducing bruising and swelling, and she gave me one for my mom. I'd moved my mom up to New York the year before so we could live closer. Since then, her mind had slipped away even more, and now her body was giving out, too.

Millie. There she is in the bed. Does she even know I went out? Where is her mind? She cries a lot, but when I ask her why, she doesn't know. Sometimes I can distract her with chocolate ice cream although what I really want to do is hug her. When she cries like that, it breaks me open. It hurts so much. She has delirium on top of dementia, yet sometimes she is clear and bright and her quirky, quick, playful personality peeks out through the cracks.

Nurse Jennifer, my favorite one because she told me she does yoga and has a boyfriend, came in to check the vitals. My mom seemed to be in a semi-coma. She hadn't moved, spoken, or really responded in any way for nearly eight days. It seemed as if upbeat Nurse Jennifer was used to that kind of situation because she just talked to us as if everything was normal.

"Your mom has amazing skin. It's so clear and smooth."

"I know. She's always had a beautiful complexion."

"I hope I have skin like that when I'm that age. In fact, I wish I had skin like that now!"

"Well, you know, she works on it. She always taught me to use a lot of moisturizer. Her technique is to lather it on so thickly that your face is covered in white goop and then just leave it there while you walk around the house."

"And eventually it just soaks in?"

"Yeah. My mom started me on that kind of program by the time I was in junior high. In fact, we used to wash our faces with Noxzema back then. Remember that stuff?"

"Yes, totally!"

We both started laughing.

"Well, it's still not bad!" Millie's words popped up even though her eyes were still closed. I think she sensed that her opinion on this matter would be respected, confident that the testimonial of her own smooth face made the case for her expertise in this area.

"That's right, Mom."

Jennifer and I laughed again but Millie was already five feet underwater again. She can't hold her mind and I can't hold her. My husband says I have to let her go.

I can't hold her in the world if she doesn't want to be here. So I hold what I can. Her soft little hands, bruised from so many IVs, are still sporting girly pink nail polish. I rub the arnica cream on her arms, or what the nurses seem to think are pincushions for their endless needles. Dark purple and green bruises, painful-looking insults, pepper the backs of her hands and the insides of her soft old lady elbows. The texture of her arms—the same ones that she hates—is beyond soft; squishy like yogurt and totally yielding in a way that seems ultra-feminine to me.

Sitting at my mom's bedside, I am grateful for my yoga and meditation practice. My meditation practice has trained me to move mindfully—sensitively feeling the texture of my yoga mat with each Downward Dog Pose; noticing my thoughts without judgment in each detoxifying deep twist; softening into a stretch rather than straining. As I stroke my mom's hair and spoon-feed her tiny bites of applesauce, I realize that these delicate moments are what I've been practicing for all these years.

Millie's been out of the hospital for ten days. She still can't get out of a chair without help and she is barely shuffling along with her walker. Two weeks in a hospital bed takes a lot out of an eighty-five-year-old and we expect it will be a couple of months before she is moving well again. But I'm proud of her and I say, "Mom, you are amazing! We're all so happy that you've improved so much. You look fantastic!" She smiles a little bit but then frowns and makes a slight gesture toward her lap. "Well, these pants don't go with this top; it's really not a great outfit."

———— •◆• ————

"Is your mother narcissistic?" Without waiting for my reply, Christiane Northrup answered for me. "Of course."

Squatting on the edge of my bed, knees in armpits, wearing distinctly non-sexy sleepwear of a tank top and baggy sweats, I pondered this question without answering. It was eight A.M. in California, eleven A.M. in Maine, and I was on the speakerphone with America's favorite women's doctor and one of my personal idols. I was hoping my tape recorder was actually recording, and even more, that I'd be able to pull off an intelligent conversation with her this early on a Monday morning.

Over the weekend I'd attended the I Can Do It! conference organized by the self-help publisher Hay House in San Diego. David had a gig at the conference playing guitar with the popular kirtan singer Krishna Das, and I piggybacked my way onto the trip. Dr. Northrup was one of the speakers and the only person I've ever known who offers a bathroom break midway through her lectures. She refers to the bathroom as "her office" since she ends up taking so many questions while waiting for a stall. She schmoozed with everybody, easily flowing from questions about vaginas to "Where did you get that pink blazer?" I noodled my way up to the stage and shyly introduced myself. Even though she was friendly and open, I felt stiff and self-conscious.

Two days later David and I drove up the coast to Los Angeles. I was thrilled that Dr. Northrup had agreed to talk to me one-on-one, but I felt nervous about the interview. I wanted to loosen up and be more myself and I decided the best way to do that was to prepare. On Monday evening I climbed up on our big hotel bed overlooking Santa Monica beach and started to bone up for the interview.

I spread out all of Dr. Northrup's major works—best-selling titles such as *Women's Bodies, Women's Wisdom; Mother-Daughter Wisdom;* and *The Secret Pleasures of Menopause*—but somehow I got sucked into *The Secret Pleasures of Menopause*. It's not what you think. It's not about avoiding hot flashes or learning to become an awesome and powerful crone now that you are over fifty. No, none of that. It's about nitric oxide and lubrication.

Dr. Northrup says bodies—like all machines—work best when lubricated. The best way to get our organs lubricated is to experience pleasure, which naturally increases blood flow, which in turn brings nutrients to your cells and removes toxins. She likens it to "stocking the fridge and emptying the garbage at the same time." And it's a natural thing that happens when we experience pleasure or feel relaxed or healthy (think sex, think yoga, think fresh air, think laughter) because of a little gas that gets released called nitric oxide. She has dedicated the second part of her life to helping women learn about everything that "can go right" in their bodies and her number-one recommendation is pleasure! What a perfect person to talk to about my body issues. Maybe she could help me learn how to turn this thing around and in turn, help my students, my friends, and women everywhere.

With high hopes and jittery nerves, I hovered over the phone on the bedside table and looked out at the ocean, trying to stay calm by breathing in and out evenly. I needn't have worried. As soon as she answered the phone, my nerves dissolved. Dr. Northrup is light, bright, outrageous, bawdy, super smart, and such a good talker! I love that she said the word *pussy* within the first fifteen minutes of our call. But before that, she covered her Uranus-Saturn conjunction in mid-heaven, local politics in Maine, and quoted Deepak Chopra, saying, "You're either part of the universal field of energy or you're not. If you are not, try to step outside of it." Then she exploded with laughter saying, "Of course, you can't!"

As our laughter died down, I confessed to her that I'd really loved her talk on Saturday. I told her how strongly I related to everything she'd said. "It's like you've been following me around my whole life!"

She wasn't surprised by this comment. "It's an interesting thing. In my astrological chart, there's something I have that exactly matches that of the entire culture. Which means what's happening in my personal life is reflective of what's happening collectively for a lot of people. And so, I pay attention to my personal life and talk about it, because it will be relevant for the collective, for many people. My whole life I've known how to talk about what was going on for me personally, not because it's personal, but because it's really important for the teaching, the healing work.

"One of the things I was taught in medical school, and I think this came from some scientific paper in the fifties, is that in the tradition of science, for most of human history, you would write down your observations using the personal pronoun 'I' as in 'This is what I found.' Somewhere in the forties or fifties, they decided that approach was 'not objective' and the personal pronoun needed to be removed."

And here she changed her voice to emphasize how ridiculous this next idea was: "As though we could separate our consciousness from what we're observing."

To illustrate the point further and to do what she does so well, combining science and medicine with soulfulness and gut wisdom, she continued: "The Heisenberg uncertainty principle states that when we observe something, we change it. That's just science. It's a scientific fact that the observer interacts with what is observed and that leads to a change in the experimental design. But they decided—whoever 'they' are—that we needed to separate ourselves from ourselves.

"All that to say, when we talk about anything including scientific studies or anything, we have to include ourselves as part of the vibration that's creating the reality. So it comes back down to—which to me is a huge relief—if you want to make a change in the planet, work on yourself.

"The beauty of my approach, I think, is that it's manageable. You work on yourself and see what happens. What a relief. You know, it's very female. It seems that the male thing is to be disembodied.

"I don't know if you ever read *The Right Stuff* by Tom Wolfe. It's about fighter pilots crashing at the beginning of the space age. As they were augering in, they would report on what the instruments were saying—'I did this and I did that.' Somewhere in their mind they knew they were about to crash and burn, but they were reporting objectively from the front, and to do that you have to separate yourself from yourself. A right-handed, left-hemisphere-dominant, white male is good at that, and it's very useful. But, for healing your body, it's deadly."

Speaking of bodies and healing, we very naturally meandered over to the subject of yoga and being embodied. That's when I finally told her I was writing a book about how I hate my body. In an instant, Christiane was off and running.

"I believe you've touched on the core issue for women, and that is, we have learned to Hate. Our. Own. Flesh.

"It comes in part from the way that the patriarchal religions have brainwashed us. I love that you're a yoga teacher because you've been steeped in the tradition that somehow we need to transcend the body. The body is a fundamental problem in most every religious text."

This struck a familiar chord. Minister's daughter learning about bodies from her minister's-wife mom . . . Yes, I would say that my mom definitely wanted to transcend her body or at least was confused by her own sexuality. For a while during my junior high years, she worked as a waitress at the diner next door to my dad's big downtown church in Seattle. The diner's owner and his wife usually ran the joint, but he got sick and so my mom stepped in to help out. She ended up staying because she liked the warm, family vibe, not to mention getting to see my dad at lunch every day and making a few extra bucks.

But one night at dinner I remember her telling my dad about

a customer who had upset her. I was only about thirteen, so I wasn't sure I really understood the problem, but from what I gathered, a man had come in for a piece of pie and, in the process, flirted with my mom. He specifically mentioned her beautiful legs. Was that a bad thing? Evidently so. Was the man creepy for saying that? Evidently so. Was my mom in danger? Maybe. Then why did I also feel like my mom was bragging a little bit, too? Even while she was telling my dad what happened, she was turning red and kerflumping. I wasn't sure if she had gotten scared or mad, or was it my dad who was mad? I think I remember him cautioning her in some kind of patronizing, protective-man way. Personally, I thought my mom was totally beautiful, including her legs. And I was pretty sure my dad thought so, too. But the whole thing translated into a message that being noticed and appreciated for your body was wrong.

At the same time that memory popped up, I responded to Christiane, "Yeah, well, I got over that transcending-the-body aspect of yoga philosophy a long time ago."

In a low just-between-me-and-you voice, she said, "Yeah, I bet you did."

I mean, I think I did. Wasn't I a child of the sixties, after all? I might have been embarrassed to show off my naked body, but that didn't make me a judgmental prude. And even if I did have a touch of sexual shyness back in the day, my new life as an NYC dancer unceremoniously gave that attitude a grand battement all the way back to Seattle.

The first time I went to Simone Forti's contact improv class in a dark and dusty Soho loft, I asked another dancer for directions to the changing room. Pulling his pants off right in front

of me, he said, "Well, I guess you can go over there in the corner if you want some privacy." I also remember Simone giving
an instruction that involved her touching her crotch, which she
called "my sex." That was also new. My teachers in California
did not use the word *sex* in dance class. So I went along, pretending these liberated attitudes were normal to me and, eventually, they were . . . sort of.

"Yogananda." I heard Christiane pulling a book off a shelf on
the other end of the line. "He's got stuff in here that you can't
believe on worldly pleasures. It's like 'please help me recover
from my sexuality.'" She took a breath. "Here we go." She read:
"'Teach me not to engross myself in passing pleasures. Teach me
to discipline my senses that they may always make me really
happy. Teach me to substitute for flesh temptation the greater
evolvement of soul happiness.'"

Like an aha moment, she cried, "There it is, right there! Of
course we hate our flesh, because we have been taught that the
downfall of humanity came because of a woman's body. Where
else would we go from there other than hating our flesh?"

By this point, I was feeling elated from this phone call. It was
massively validating to know that my hero, Christiane Northrup,
immediately found this topic so discussion worthy. In fact, she
was positioning the whole women-body-self-esteem issue as a
fulcrum for women: Change yourself and change the world.
That fit in perfectly with my bodhisattva ideal, which was kind
of funny considering where she next took the conversation—
out of the spiritual and into the street.

"I was on the *Rachael Ray Show*, booked to talk about
the female erogenous anatomy inside the pelvis. I was waiting in

the green room with the other guests, including several women, ages twenty-four to probably fifty-five, who were complaining about finding good men. I said, 'I could take you out on the streets of Manhattan and find you a date.' The producers called me later and said, 'Could you do that?' I said, 'I could, but I'm not going to, because right here in Manhattan is the master from whom I learned—Regena Thomasauer.' Mama Gena teaches flirting as a spiritual exercise at her School of Womanly Arts. She says it's the art of enjoying yourself in the company of another. That's all. It's not to get anything. It's simply to uplift the moment."

Here she paused to let this concept sink in. I loved the idea that we can enjoy our bodies and engage in flirting, not to get anything, but simply to feel joy and hot energy and to raise everyone's spirits. This was another new idea for me. Or was it? Isn't that what we were doing for Larry Kirwan on his birthday in the St. Marks Bar?

I started to say something, but Christiane had already raced ahead. "Mama Gena told the women that the first step is to find a man who is not dangerous, and go up to him. You don't have to make eye contact or anything. But you begin to admire something about him, maybe his hands, maybe his hair. Whatever.

"And while you do"—another pause to make sure I was ready for this—"you think about your pussy!" She loved telling me this. "I know, it's outrageous, but in that one moment, it all came together for me. Oh. My. God. All the power of those old caves shaped like vaginas and covered with triangles—it's not that we're supposed to go back to that time when the female body was seen as sacred. We can do it right now!

"So, for the *Rachael Ray Show,* Regena took three women in

their forties out to a drinking establishment in the Wall Street area. Before going up to the bar, she took them into the ladies' room to take off their underwear. Obviously you can't say 'pussy' on national television, even though you can talk about the female erogenous anatomy inside the pelvis! So, Mama Gena called it 'their business.' Think about your business."

Here was another point she wanted me to hear loud and clear. "The trick is that energy follows awareness. The female anatomy is where the magic is. We've been talked out of it. But it's where the magic is.

"And in the yogic tradition, we're always trying to transcend our desires. Guess what? That's a desire!

"As long as you're on earth, you're going to have desires. Where are you going to feel them? In your body. How are you going to know that you're on the right track? You feel it in your genitals. Woo hoo! So we're taught our whole lives, don't go there."

It's the old starving-Buddha-in-the-forest story, only she's flipped it on its head. Yeah, desire comes from the body, but instead of denying the body, we accept the body. We appreciate the body and even love the body. The lesson is definitely that whatever happens, stay embodied and aware. Where was she when I was a little girl? As I'm wondering that, Christiane is already going there.

"Oh, and by the way, I was showing the guy in my life a video of Regena taking the women into the bar. She gives them mantras—'I am gorgeous'—things you say in your head before doing something scary.

"And the guy says to me, 'I don't understand. You've known

this since you were a little girl.' and I said, 'No, I haven't.' It's like my guy thinks that somehow women know they have this power. They don't! And I couldn't convince him that they don't. He said every woman knows this. That's why they're told not to speak to strangers." She agreed with that part. "You're told that before you have your frontal lobe intellect on board. You don't even know that something is bad or wrong with your body."

I thought back again to Larry Kirwan's birthday party. We wanted to be brave and bold, but we were pretending, even to ourselves. We were supposedly giving him a present, yet we all held something back. Maybe we couldn't give it all away because of the primal patterning we'd received as girls—that giving ourselves was actually having something taken from us. I wondered what Christiane thought about that, so I said, "And then if you let anybody go to that place with you, you'll lose something."

Of course, she got that right away. "You'll lose something— right! You are allowing this person into the sanctum sanctorum. This is the source of God—right here. This is the quickest way to God Realization, when you understand the connection between spirituality and sexuality."

Inspired but overwhelmed, I asked, "So how do we keep on the track with that? Because it seems like the negative thinking patterns that have been implanted are so powerful. Is there a path toward shifting the balance?"

"The beauty is that's what happening right now on the planet. A woman sent me a Facebook link called Sex, Chocolate, and Your Pelvic Floor. I clicked on it and found that in Texas they're doing these wonderful pelvic floor exercises and the women are starting to own their Shakti, their divine feminine power. Usually you can only do this in a group. A woman alone, it's really scary. But when you get women together, they get really bawdy really quickly. They just go right there, and it's hilarious because women egg each other on."

"And we've been waiting so long." Why did I say that? By we, did I really mean me?

She was nice enough not to say that. "Yes, we've been waiting, so now it's happening. I believe this is where we're going. It's where we have to go—being that bawdy, wonderful Shakti."

I loved that she was talking my yoga language. *Yoga* means the "union of opposites." It says that we all have feminine and masculine energies. The divine feminine power of Shakti is just as essential as divine male power, but has different qualities. Shakti is about creation, fertility, change, liberation. Naturally, Shakti is most manifest in female bodies. Consciously tapping into this energy invites a big whoosh of earthy-body bawdiness to rise up from the cave-like power spot between a woman's legs, "her sex."

The subject of bawdiness brings Christiane back to Mama Gena. "At first I thought Regena was a nut bag. What kind of woman runs around in a pink feather boa?"

"I have a pink feather boa," I said, and then my voice faded a bit, "but it's in the back of my closet."

"Well, yeah." Her voice said it all, and I got the message. You may have the feather boa, Cyndi, but clearly it/you are still in the closet. But then she started to give me advice, which was the reason I had wanted to talk to her in the first place. I strained to open my ears wider.

"You have to have a sense of humor about it. I have this fabulous little tango top that came with some Tango Babe clothes. It was perfect for this woman I know who also dances tango. So I gave it to her. She's just adorable. She's about fifty and of course, she doesn't know that she has a perfect body and is gorgeous. So I gave it to her and she said, 'I could never wear that. Never!'

"I said, 'Okay, could you wear it in the bathroom? Look at yourself in the mirror? Just look at that Tango Babe logo and say, "I'm a Tango Babe"?'

"She said, 'I don't know. I don't think so.' I said, 'Could you try it at least once?'

"And then she's talking about how uptight she is, and she says, 'I am so stupid. I am so bad,' and I said, 'You can say "I'm so stupid. I'm so bad," but then why don't you say, "How adorable is that?" That's what you have to do. You have to take the Nazi in your head and put a feather boa on it.'"

Whoa. That was the best piece of advice I'd ever heard. I'm not even sure I understood what it meant exactly, but I was certainly familiar with that inner drill sergeant.

"It's the only way. Nothing else works. Because remember the old feminist adage, 'the father's house will never be dismantled by the father's tools.' You're not going to be able to fight your body hatred with the left hemisphere, with the intellect that's always judging and cutting and all the rest of it. You can never do it that way. You have to come in from the right hemisphere, and the right hemisphere has connections to the body. You have to go back to being a silly girl."

Looking back now, I cannot believe that this amazing,

brilliant piece of advice seemed to go in one of my ears and out the other, but it did. Perhaps it was too deep, too juicy, too overwhelming. It was exactly the advice I needed to hear, but somehow I couldn't take it in. For a while yet, I would still be in my head, labeling thoughts but not really feeling them; not allowing my energy to drop down to the warm cave of my heart or my Shakti. So for now, I just changed the subject.

I asked her, "One thing that you talked about on Saturday was biologic age versus chronologic age. That was interesting to me because I can stand on my head and do all kinds of great things, but there is a little voice that's starting to say, 'You know, you don't look bad for fifty-six.' You talked about the notion of self-limiting. Is there a way to accept your age without being self-limiting?"

Gracious as always, she replied, "You simply have to decide that age is irrelevant. I have come to the conclusion that ageism is the last big ism that's acceptable. Racism is not acceptable and classism is not acceptable, nor is sexism, but ageism is acceptable. You'll see people who are eighty-five and in nursing homes saying, 'I don't want to be around those old people.'"

With a knowing tone, I said, "My mother."

"She doesn't want to be around those other people, right?"

"Right, and yet she's completely out of it. She has Lewy body. Her mind and her body are messed up, but she's still doesn't want to be around those other people. And she's proud of being the best-looking woman there, with the nicest clothes."

Without realizing it, I've just given Christiane something really juicy to bite into. Even though she was theoretically the

interviewee, she was listening closely to everything I said.
When she heard me describe my mom, she had another understanding about me and the whole topic of female bodies.

She was clear about declaring my mom narcissistic, but I
hesitated to chime in my agreement. I felt so bad about my
mom, I couldn't bear to say anything critical about her. But then
I did. "I think she is," I said quietly.

Christiane did not hesitate. "I know she is or she wouldn't be
saying that." Her energy had spiked up again. The doctor was
on! "So! You are the daughter of a narcissistic mother. You can
never be good enough when you have a narcissistic mother,
because she has an abyss inside and no sense of self. No amount
of external validation can fill that abyss inside her."

"Yeah, you just totally nailed it."

"I'm a bit narcissistic as well," she continued. "I'm one of that
group."

Even though she was leading the way, I was not ready to
stick that label on myself, so I waffled. "I guess I'm kind of
that way."

"Well, yeah." Her tone implied that this was obvious. "Because
our bodies were created within that consciousness, you see."
Was that my genetic inheritance? Did I catch my mother's narcissism while I was still in the womb?

Okay, I admit my mother and I are akin in this way as well.
But still, I qualified my admission by insisting I really didn't want
to be that way anymore. I've realized that being so self-focused
is not healthy and that I want to change. "So what should I do?"
I asked.

"You've been proving yourself and you've been surviving. Now, for you, it's all about thriving. About age fifty-nine, sixty is when life really begins. You don't take anything seriously anymore. It's a very exciting time."

Her voice got loud again to make her point: "From now on you have to be led by life force. You have to be led by Shakti, or everything will disintegrate."

Then she got quiet. "You know that."

"Yes, I can feel that," I replied. "I don't want to be shut off from my life force anymore, not just for myself but for every woman. I'm a yoga teacher and a lot of people are looking to me." I just had to throw that in so that she knew that even though I might lean toward narcissism, I'm not selfish.

She heard that. She heard it all and framed her next bit of advice around my bodhisattva bent, reminding me that what's good for me is good for everybody.

"The lighter you can become, the more open, the more luscious, the more giggling, the better for everyone. I want you to experience what I call the 'placenta of Shakti.'"

There was that word *light* again. And Shakti. That had come up for me before, too. "I've been told by an Ayurvedic astrologer/palm reader that I'm sitting on a volcano of Shakti."

Christiane said, "Yes, but it hasn't been time. Now it is time. You had to create a sturdy foundation. The Shakti, as you know, can blow you right out. That's why they say the tantric path has the most bodies littered along the way. But you have the discipline. That's important. Now the Shakti has a strong container and that's what the rest of your life is going to be."

————— • ◆ • —————

A few months later, I traveled back to India, the ancestral home of Shakti, the goddess of creative female energy.

Smith has told me that after a day of traveling it is natural to gain weight and feel bloated. He says it's just water weight from sitting so long. In my case, it might be more than that. The fifteen-hour flight to India started out fine. David and I were ecstatic about our upgrade to first class. Holding hands as we reclined in the sexy pod-like seating, we said yes to everything on offer, starting with a champagne toast to ourselves to celebrate our first trip to India together.

But just as the curried shrimp appetizers were arriving, the pilot's voice interrupted our movie to announce that we were going to experience some turbulence. He tried to downplay it by mentioning that this particular hurricane had just been downgraded to a tropical storm and by speaking in that mid-American twang that is meant to suggest the pilot is actually a cowboy and completely in control. None of that was reassuring. What reassures me when I'm flying over the ocean in a huge tin can that is bucking and rocking side to side is a glass of wine. Perhaps even a few glasses of wine. With every *kerplunk* I could just feel my cortisol going through the roof! You'd think with all the flying I do I'd be used to it, but I'm not and I know self-medicating is denial in action, but it's the only thing that keeps me in my skin at times like that. The bumps didn't last too long and I really didn't drink too much, but the next day I woke up in India feeling fat, fat, fat. Again.

How did this happen? Two years after my first pilgrimage

through India, here I am again. Back on a bus with no shocks, riding through the mountains of Darjeeling, and once again obsessing about how tight my waistband feels. These pants were comfortable four days ago when I was packing for this trip. But now as I bounced along the mountain roads of Sikkim, I felt miserable, disgusted, and frustrated and full of negative thoughts about myself coupled with those same old boring vows to eat less, eat different, exercise more.

A few days later I felt good again. I'd gotten over my jet lag a bit and after three bed-buggy hotels offering cold, watery porridge and cold-water showers, we'd checked into the Mayfair Gangtok—a shiny new hotel spa and casino that was a Sikkimese cross between Las Vegas and Disneyland. Around every corner of the maze-like complex we discovered bigger-than-life-size, rainbow-colored Buddha statues similar to the inspiring ones I'd seen in Deer Park, only these statues were done in high-gloss varnish, along with splashy fake waterfalls and real Hindu fire altars with real Hindu monks chanting real Hindu chants.

The hotel entrance welcomed us with a kneeling Garuda statue—the ancient birdman with a beak-like nose, regal crown, and large red wings. He is said to be a mythical protector and was, I thought, a charming balance to the more earthly armed guards and metal detectors. But those were signs of the modernity of this hotel and also meant that our bedroom floor was sparkly, clean wood and perfect for yoga.

Instead of replaying the same soap opera that arises over a mere five pounds, I brought to mind Collette's words about the feminine nature of waxing and waning. I remembered Jamie's five-pound window. I reminded myself that these new five

pounds were impermanent. I reviewed the definition of meditation as a "placing of attention." In fact, we are always placing our
attention on something, but meditation is a conscious placing of
it, or perhaps an un-placing of attention, away from things that
don't need more attention.

My old mental habits had been strong, but little by little, just
like yoga, my meditation practice was weakening them. Even
though it felt comfortable to berate myself, I recognized that I'd
been there before and it felt like old news. This time, perhaps
feeling safe in the mandala of Garuda or close to the energy
bank of Shakti, I was inspired to keep my commitment to expanding my comfort zone by doing something different, something beneficial.

So, after a hot shower and a nap, I got down on my hands
and knees, and reconnected to my body in a positive way. That
sounds sexy and it was definitely sensuous. I started with a few
cat and cow stretches to warm up my spine, then worked my
way into a delicious Downward Dog Pose. Feeling energized, I
rolled up to standing and moved into some powerful, strengthening Warrior Poses.

Inspired by my friend at the front gate, I did a Garudasana,
which is a balancing pose with one leg wrapped around the
other, arms intertwined in front of my face. When I teach this
pose to my students, I always tell them that the inner quality of
the Garuda is said to be Outrageous. The Garuda is outrageous
because, although it is a flying being, it never lands. It never
lands because it never gets tired. It never gets tired because it
rides the wind. I take a deep breath in, remembering that the
wind is my breath. When I resist the way things are going, I feel

bad. This is not the same as surrendering or being weak. But it does mean that when I look at things as they are and work with the situation at hand, I am more likely to make positive choices that make me feel more grounded, healthy, and connected to myself and my life. I exhaled for eight slow counts.

Okay, Garudasana on the other leg and then down onto my back for some much-needed spinal twisting to detox my inner organs and soften up my back muscles that had been gripping like mad on that bus.

I finished my practice with my favorite pose, called Legs Up the Wall Pose. I bounced sideways onto the cushy, clean bed and then swung my legs like a mermaid's tail up onto the headboard, just below a gold spray-painted Buddha print. I felt myself relax as the lymph and water in my legs reversed, de-swelling my ankles and feet. I love this pose because even though it is completely easy and absolutely anybody can do it, almost anywhere, anytime, it is extremely good for you. One of the most beneficial results of this asana is that because you are upside down, your heart has to work a little bit harder than usual to pump your blood. So even though you are just lying there doing nothing, your heart is getting stronger. A very friendly ratio of effort to reward. In almost every way, Legs Up the Wall Pose is a rebalancing, including that it is a restorative yoga pose. Once I was comfortably situated on the bed, a few fluffy pillows under my pelvis and a small throw folded under my head, my job was to just lie there and be open to the experience. This is the feminine aspect of yoga, the receptive element, which reminds us that sometimes doing less brings the most positive results.

By the next morning my digestion was back on track, and

when I looked in the full-length mirror, my spirits lifted. I looked and felt much lighter and I felt pleased with myself for energetically embracing my body, instead of getting stuck in my head's habitual stew of frustration.

As I got dressed in those cute purple pants, which fit perfectly once again, I recognized this whole drama as a very familiar roller coaster. When my body is in balance, my mind functions better and I feel upbeat and positive. It strikes me that my life walks a pretty delicate tightrope if my buttons are so easily pushed by something that is always going to change—the ebb and flow of tides in my personal aquifer.

But bit by bit, my mindfulness practice was proving effective. I felt some space opening in my mind, some kindness coming in, some willingness not to react in the same old way. I know in my heart that this is how suffering decreases, not necessarily in a sudden flash of awakening, but breath by breath by breath.

Before getting back on the bus for another bumpy forty-mile ride that would take at least four hours, I pulled one of the scarlet satin cushions off the glitzy love seat in our room. I wiggled my butt around on it for a few moments until I felt settled and grounded. I placed my attention on my breath and sat quietly. No need to rush to the bus yet. No need to fill space with activity, in body or mind, when receptivity will do. I just sat and breathed and when my mind strayed, I gently returned it to my breath.

———— ◆ ————

While I was in India, Millie developed a life-threatening bedsore. She would need skilled nursing care going forward, and so

I moved her to a new facility and hired Maureen, a nurses' aide/
personal companion to bathe her, dress her, feed her, and keep
her safe. Feeling comfortable with me, Maureen didn't bother to
say hi when I walked into my mom's room at the nursing home.
She just looked up at me and said, "Now see, if I had a figure like
that, I'd be showing it off!" I looked down at what I was wearing
and my mind went blank. First of all, I thought it was a pretty
tight sweater already; and second, I don't think my figure is that
great, not to mention that I was having an I-feel-fat day. But
there was no way that I'm going to say anything like that to
Maureen, and anyway, she might be right. She has a great sense
of style and I love how she looked in her tomato-gold-and-
green-striped blouse, sparkly stretch pants, green eye shadow,
orange lipstick, and blond wig.

It only took two days after she first started working for my
mom for Maureen to tell me the story of her body. I never asked
her anything about it, but we were both sitting by my mom's
bed for hours and just naturally got to talking about the kinds
of things that women talk about when they're getting to know
each other. Hair, skin, bodies. She wasn't wearing her wig that
day and I discovered we both have gray hair. That broke the ice.
Then Maureen told me that she hadn't always been at her current size; in fact, she had lost one hundred fifty pounds about
eight years back. She did it by walking four hours a day for a
year and a half. Two hours in the morning to get to work and
two hours coming back home.

Now that I know how hard she works I am even more
impressed. Maureen is the primary caretaker for my mom. She
works twelve-hour shifts, eight A.M. to eight P.M., mostly

unsupervised. She doesn't need anybody to tell her what to do because she is a trained nurse's aide, she has an impeccable work ethic, and mostly she is an angel. She cares. She is extra kind to me, too, because she knows my heart is breaking a little more every day as my mom diminishes. We found out today that my mom weighs eighty-two pounds.

But Maureen? Well, she gained those one hundred fifty pounds back and more. She can just barely squeeze down into the arms of the bedside chair. I've never seen her eat anything (which we all know is usually a sign of secret bingeing) but she doesn't have a chance to get much exercise these days either. She has to take a couple of buses and a train to get to the nursing home by eight A.M. and doesn't make it back home until around ten thirty. No time to walk.

She says to me, "You must eat really healthy."

"Well, I try to." And then I feel guilty because I know that I do sometimes have dessert or corn chips and guacamole or red wine.

Maureen says, "I'd like to eat healthier, but fast food is less expensive." And then I feel sad, and I wonder if I can afford to give Maureen a raise.

Maureen says, "You must do a lot of yoga to get such a nice figure."

"Well, but, there is always this bit of fat around my waist that I can't seem to get rid of."

Oops. For a moment I thought Maureen and I were like me and my other friends, all the friends I've had since junior high. We were not raised in a way that allowed us to understand the confidence of the seventy-year-old woman in Lola's store. Women who did that were considered arrogant at best and, more likely, sluts. So I naturally went to a self-critical place. But then I realized Maureen and I are not in the same body ballpark, so I stopped squeezing my spare tire and instead I said, "Yes, I do yoga most every day and it's fun! I'll give you a free pass to come to my yoga studio." She chuckled and it really did look like she was sitting in a bucket of Jell-O.

"Maureen, you could start in the Brand New Beginners class where everyone feels self-conscious at first and nobody is in shape or knows anything about yoga."

Her response to that is a combo of a sweet smile and a head tilt that says, "Are you kidding?" She doesn't have to tell me with words that she wouldn't be caught dead walking into a yoga studio with that body.

So I say, "I will give you a video and you can do it at home."

She laughs and says, "I have a video and I like to watch it while I eat!"

"Well, that's a start, I guess!" We both crack up.

I try another approach. Sitting up nice and straight, on the edge of the seat I say, "Well, you know what, Maureen? Yoga doesn't have to be a big deal. Really. Just whenever you think of it and since you are sitting here for hours anyway, you can take a deep breath in"—I demonstrate by sitting up even taller and drawing in a long, full inhalation—"and then, as you exhale, do a little twist." I carefully place my left hand on my right thigh and my right arm on the back of the chair. Then I do a small twist, as if I also had a very large body so that Maureen will get the idea that this simple chair yoga exercise is completely available to her right now, just as she is. But when I untwist I see that

Maureen is just looking at me. She is staring at me but she is not following my instructions.

"You can also try breathing exercises right in your chair. Try this." As I lift my arms up I say, "Inhale, one, two, three, four."

Maureen does not move.

"And exhale, arms down, one, two, three, four."

Laughing again, she pushes down hard on the arms of the chair to haul herself up onto her perpetually swollen feet. "There is no way that I am going to do that in front of anyone."

But now Maureen has stopped listening to me. She is bending over my tiny mom, softly rubbing Vaseline on her lips. She bathes my mom every day, taking care with her feet where the skin is especially thin. She combs her hair and brushes her teeth with a Q-tip. She gently squirts Ensure between her lips with a turkey baster.

Maureen keeps busy all day long, turning my mom from side to side, picking her up and putting her in her wheelchair, getting her to accept one more spoonful of soup, wiping away any dribbles or crumbs on her bib.

Maureen takes care of my mom as if she were her very precious cargo, but like so many other women, she doesn't have time to take care of herself.

———— ✦ ————

Beginning yoga students almost always respond the same way to an instruction that they've never heard before. Perhaps they are in a familiar, stable lunge position, right leg forward and left leg extended long behind them, both hands firmly planted on the floor. So far they've been following along with my verbal instructions, but when I say, "Now, tuck your right shoulder behind your right knee," they stop in their tracks. Some of them simply sit down. Others not only stop what they are doing, but look at me like I'm crazy. "What?" they might say, or "No way!" The new instruction doesn't compute, so they basically freak out.

Advanced students react to unpredictable directives in the opposite way; their responses generally fall into one of two categories. They receive the instruction and simply give it a try. Or they may pause in mid-position/action and take a moment to consider. From that gap in time and space, they slowly start to wriggle their shoulder behind their knee. If that doesn't work, they might lift their front hip a bit to create more room for their shoulder, take hold of the back of their ankle to create some leverage and then try it again. It's fun for them to puzzle out this new instruction.

The beginners are coming from a goal-oriented perspective. They only hear an end-point position, which they immediately interpret as something out of the realm of their possibility—as if I had said, levitate into the air and hover at ten feet. They assume they can't do it because they haven't done it before and probably have never seen anyone else do it.

As the teacher, I may need to give them a demonstration but first I like to give the instruction and see how they respond. My job is to lead the students through clear, precise, and appropriate instruction. I create "dots" for them all along the way, but the real learning begins when they start to make their own connections.

This is what we talk about more than the actual yoga pose and it is the teaching that I think is most valuable. At the end of the day, who cares if you can put your shoulder behind your knee? But if you've strengthened your ability to listen well, cultivated curiosity in possibilities, and developed some confidence in your own wisdom, then you've really made a shift that is useful. This process is what we are practicing in yoga class.

The advanced students have already learned about the meaning of practice. They've embodied the knowledge that if they stay steady, stick with the process, and keep moving along, even if they are unsure of both the path and the destination, eventually the way will become clear. They learn to be comfortable with problem solving and, in fact, understand that that is a lot of what yoga or meditation or any kind of mindfulness practice is really about. Taking a look at any given situation and working with things as they are. Not just, how can this position turn into that position? But what is the process of transition for turning this position into that position, with this body (tight hips, weak knees, strong shoulders) and this mind (curious, clear, foggy, scattered) right now? Is there friction involved? Yes. The yoga word for friction is *tapas*, which really means that where there is heat, there is the potential for transformation.

For the super advanced students, this is where the practice begins. They are most interested in friction because that's where the alchemy takes place.

———— • ◆ • ————

"Just thought you might want to know what people are saying about you." An email from a guy I'd met only once, ten years earlier in Germany, but of course, it was easy to find me through Facebook. He wanted to let me know that a former student of mine had moved back to her home in Berlin and had just published a memoir of her time in NYC, a dishy tell-all about the yoga gossip she'd uncovered. Wouldn't I want to know about her published claim that "a friend of mine" who taught meditation classes had been involved in some "unsavory" activities? In less time than it takes to even have a thought, I had a sick feeling in my stomach. It was also a knowing feeling; I knew the unnamed "friend" was my husband.

I took a deep breath and shook off that bad feeling. What could I do about it right then, and anyway, I had to go teach a yoga class. But that night I showed my husband. "Look at this weird email I got today, David." I read it to him, and he instantly freaked out. Generally David is measured in his responses, good at seeing both sides of things and not quick to judge. So when he had this over-the-top response—"That's outrageous! Who is she anyway? I want to see this book! I want an exact translation! This is libel!"—I knew instantly that it was about him. The bad feeling was back.

I've learned to listen to feelings in my body, as another form of meditation practice. Often when I'm walking home from the studio, I'll realize that I have a butterfly in my stomach or I'm gripping the strap of my yoga bag too hard. I practice being curious about it. It's fun. I investigate by asking myself, "Okay, what's bothering me?" The answer is usually right there on the surface and then I can puzzle it through, either coming to a resolution or at least gaining enough awareness of the issue to be able to table it for now and bookmark it for later. The body knows, the mind clarifies, and when I can get them to hold hands with my breath, things usually work out all right.

A couple of days later I realized that bad feeling—an eating-away kind of feeling as if I'd had way too much coffee—was still there. I'd been ignoring it, which is not the same as bookmarking something for later. It's denial and it will eat away at you.

So I brought up the subject again, and again I was met with the same reaction from him and the same knowing inside me.

"Really?" I asked. "You really don't know anything about this? Because if there is something true here I'd prefer to hear it from you."

He sat back in his chair with a sigh and confessed that at times, he had gone to "gentlemen's clubs" without wanting me to know. With that new information, off I went to teach a class.

That night at dinner he was especially gracious to me; standing up when I entered the restaurant and holding out my chair; his gentlemanly elegance on full display. He said he understood that I might feel slimed; that of course I would feel bad about the deception and so did he. I said it was really no big deal but I didn't know why I said that. I didn't really know what I thought, but I still knew what I felt: bad, coffee acid, icky.

When I woke up the next morning I was surprised to have the feeling still lingering. Somehow I knew there must be more. Once again I asked for his consideration: "Please don't let me find out anything else through Facebook, okay?"

He took a hard look at me. "Do you really think you can handle the truth?"

"Go ahead."

And then he told me about other women, several affairs, things I had never thought would ever happen in my marriage.

Whoa. I didn't see that coming. It knocked the breath out of me. I was so shocked that everything turned to liquid inside me and I had to run to the bathroom. I came back to the living room feeling very shaky. I sat on the couch and waited.

He said that if I had been a more loving, more attentive wife, it wouldn't have happened.

He said he's always loved my body, always thought I was beautiful. Hadn't he always told me that? But, he said, I just didn't hear him and instead hid myself from him.

He said, "What do you expect? You're the one who's writing a book about how you hate your body."

He said that I'd been obsessed with taking care of my mother, my business, even my dog—everything and everyone but him.

Was he right? It's true that I had been overwhelmed with the care needs of my mother. And yes, my business is also demanding. Clearly I hadn't been caring for David in the way he wanted, but I couldn't abandon my mother, could I? She has no one else. I had to take care of her. And I couldn't abandon my business, and who else would take the dog to the vet, and he might think I didn't take care of him, but that's because men just don't notice all the things you do for them at home, right?

The coffee feeling in my stomach was gone now, replaced by a global feeling of pain and exhaustion. And then, I had to get up, put on my yoga clothes, walk up the street to my studio, and lead my teacher-training group. Thirty minutes after this revelation, feeling shaky, I started the class by ringing the gong for a mindfulness meditation session.

And there I sat. It was hard not to cry but that wasn't the time or place. My body felt really weird, clammy and stressed. My mind was like the spin cycle, thoughts flying everywhere as

I tried to understand that what I'd just heard was not a dream. It was real. My marriage was not what I thought it was. It was hard for me to maintain a good upright posture. I was being pulled down by a heavy feeling in my chest, which brought to life the worn-out phrase "broken heart."

All I could do was sit with that. Conceptually, I told myself that this feeling would shift, but right then it felt like this was a kind of cellular ouch that wasn't going anywhere soon.

During the lunch break, I went to my office, closed the door, and sat down on my red couch. I cried and cried and sat and cried and then a new thought arose. It occurred to me that I had gotten something wrong. It was the bodhisattva vow. In my efforts to be helpful to others, I had forgotten that this vow is supposed to be two-pronged. It's a commitment to helping all sentient beings become free and happy, *including oneself*. In fact, the teachings say that if you can't be compassionate to yourself, you can't be compassionate and caring to others. You can't be a schmuck to yourself and then be sweet to others. It just doesn't work like that. You have to start with yourself. That is the only path. There is no other way. How had I missed that essential detail?

Menopause. It's not an excuse but it is an explanation for much of what had been going on with me. In addition to grieving over my father's recent death and despairing over the loss of my mother as I knew her, while still having sole responsibility for her care, I noticed that my sexual appetite had waned over the last several years. Mentally, I cared about this. Does anyone want to think of themselves as an asexual being? When I thought of myself like that I didn't like it, but physically, I didn't care. My groin-ycologist told me later that menopause creates a catch-22 because when you have no libido you also have no motivation to get a libido. Everything in the body is interdependent; the whole system is a vinyasa, really, so when your libido tanks it is indicative of what is happening throughout the entire network of your body and mind.

All the natural elements of your energy weaken, such as water, which evaporates, leaving you with dry skin, hair, and nails; your wind energy lessens, which makes it a drag to do aerobic activity and generally leaves you in a state of less oomph. The fire element hands you a double whammy: Your digestive fires cool down, giving you that menopause belly pooch, and at the same time, your internal thermostat starts spiking, giving you unexpected rushes and flushes at the most inopportune moments. You suddenly find yourself with a sweaty brow while giving a talk in front of a group of people, or being awakened by an adrenaline rush at three o'clock in the morning. It's tough stuff.

I would try to make a little joke by gesturing toward my lap and saying, "You are dead to me!" And my husband and I would laugh, but not really. Yet there was a part of me that was okay with this new non-sensation. I remembered what I had learned in yoga philosophy about the four stages of Indian society: Youth is the time for education; early adulthood is the time for marriage and creating a family; the third phase of life is slowing down and getting your business affairs settled; and finally, one's purpose in the last stage of life is to be old and asexual, naturally turning away from lust and sensuality and devoting oneself to spiritual pursuits.

I thought about this a lot. I thought why can't I go with what feels natural and organic to me? Since turning fifty I'd been desperate to spend more time outside in nature and when I was inside, I found myself drawn to domestic activities such as knitting and making throw pillows, things I'd learned from my mom but had been too busy and active to engage in for decades. Now I was completely content to sit for hours crocheting sweaters for bottles, making cute flower vases that I gave to my girlfriends. I found this relaxing. Sex did not seem relaxing. It took effort and the other thing was, the really bad thing was, that it hurt. Nobody talks about this and so I thought that it was just me. Another wrong thing about my body.

There's another catch-22 with menopause, as well; one that is a serious trap between a rock and a hard place. Women are faced with choosing whether to take hormones and potentially up their risk of getting cancer, or trying to have painful sex, or giving up on the whole thing all together. Another option is to silently freak out and avoid dealing with it, which is what I did. I didn't know that going to the groin-ycologist is not just about getting an annual pap. I had no idea that she has lots of ways to help you feel sexual energy and arousal and attraction again. There are hormone creams and patches and small, safer doses and new kinds of tests to monitor your health all along the way. But I didn't know any of this then. I just didn't feel sexy and I didn't know what to do about it. I didn't know who to ask or how to ask. I felt embarrassed and like an Indian senior citizen, I turned away from my sensuality, letting it die a natural death.

So it was true that I hadn't given my husband the sexual attention he needed and deserved and he was right to expect more from me. But I hadn't taken care of him because I hadn't even been able to take care of myself.

Isn't the path of self-care what Jamie took when she outed herself in *More?* Didn't Christiane support that notion when she told me to go for joy and ride my Shakti? Isn't wanting goodness for yourself what Tia meant when she used the word *light?* My mindfulness practice was helping me, but it was still something going on in my head.

Crying on my red couch put me back in my body again and I knew in my gut that the root of the whole problem was that I had not been taking care of myself. I knew it because I also felt mad. I felt the tiniest little bit of protectiveness toward my own self, that self that was feeling so hurt and unseen right then. And that little seed, nestled in my second brain somewhere around my navel chakra, was trying to tell me something.

Gelek Rimpoche had taught me that the Tibetan words for mind and heart are the same: *citta.* As I remembered that, I had another knowing, more wisdom from the brain in my gut. It told me that I would get through this, that I just had to stay out of my head and stay down in my heart. And when I thought about doing that, the little seed grew a voice, which popped up and pushed itself forward, drowning out the other chattering voices expressing hurt and shock about a relationship that wasn't the safe haven I had thought it was. This voice wasn't the familiar grumpster, but came from a different, more friendly and confident place. This voice said, "There's nothing wrong with you."

Dissolving

———•◆•———

Every life and every death begins the same way, with an exhale. We come into the world with a cry and go out with a sigh, each of these expressions floating on the out-breath.

Buddha's disciple, Maudgalyayana, taught his own student an important lesson by showing him a huge pile of bones. When the student asked, "What is that?" Maudgalyayana replied, "These are all the bones from the bodies you had in previous lives."

The bones are always the first to go; it is how the earth element in our body dissolves. Water goes next, followed by the element of fire. Then our wind blows out. After the air element leaves us, the only thing left is our consciousness and finally that exits the body, too.

Some say that after forty days we are reborn. The root of the word *incarnate* means "to cause to heal." We leave our bodies behind, yet our minds become healed as we rotate through the cycle of arising, abiding, and dissolving.

We are lucky that we can embody this vinyasa without actually dying. The body that we leave behind could be the carcass of a hard idea, or the rotting frame of a destructive pattern of behavior.

We are lucky that we can practice dissolving without losing the good stuff. As we breathe out we really can just let go of all the hard thoughts, which make hard hearts. The Sanskrit word for heart is *hridayam*, which means "that which takes, circulates, and gives." Hearts are meant to be pliant; to pump; their job the ultimate "placing in a special way."

Without giving, there is no receiving. Without letting go, there is no letting in. Without dissolving, there is no new arising. Without an exhale, there is no inhale.

———•◆•———

"What's wrong with you anyway? What is it that you want? Who is not giving you the love you need?"

"I'd like to feel more love from my husband," I replied meekly.

"Well, no wonder he doesn't love you! All you do is complain and whine about your body!"

I knew I shouldn't have mentioned how I'd avoided a beach date early on in my relationship with my now-husband-then-boyfriend, because I didn't want him to see my cellulite.

What I didn't know was that this verbal slap was a portent of things to come and certainly not the kind of comment I had been expecting from Louise Hay. After all, she is famous as a goddess of the self-help movement and the birth mother of positive affirmations. Her messages of love and healing uplifted the gay community during the eighties and this work bled into the dance community, where I was first introduced to her book *You Can Heal Your Life* by a dancer friend of mine who used it to get rid of her chronic yeast infections. Although Louise claims that she used affirmations to heal her own cervical cancer, she doesn't make any other claims about curing, although she does clarify what healing means by saying that it is "not always of the body."

"Well, great!" I thought. "That means she is the perfect

person for me to talk to." I was by now heartily sick of the whole drama, more than ready to heal my life, expunge the gnawing voice eating me from the inside out, silence the James Joyce–worthy run-on sentence endlessly telling me that my body was deficient. All this, I figured, could be purged forever, just like Louise's cancer, by letting go of my body-obsessed approach and zapping the problem with a consciousness cocktail of positive mental work.

I'd met Louise previously upon the publication of OM yoga in a Box, a kit for practicing yoga at home that includes a candle, incense, a yoga strap, and flash cards, which demonstrate my instructions on the enclosed yoga class CD. I remembered her as warm and supportive. I'd been touched when she also sent me a note saying something super positive about my product, which I later figured out was an affirmation. Since then I hadn't heard from Louise Hay and I could tell she didn't remember me. The first time I'd seen her since then was the day before our talk, when she opened the I Can Do It! conference.

Yes, it is called that and not the You Can Do It! conference because this way whenever you and your girlfriend talk about your plans for going to the conference, and when you ask your boss for time off to attend this conference, and when you tell your husband you're going to this conference without him because you need to find something just for yourself, you end up saying this affirmation over and over again: I Can Do It. I Can Do It. I Can Do It. Louise never tires of helping people find ways to affirm their potential, because she knows that we have to start with ourselves. I Can Do It affirms that healing happens not by our being cheerleaders for others, but by our being cheerleaders for ourselves. So why was I so surprised that she did not want to be a cheerleader for me?

Maybe because I thought of her as a saint. The conference opened with Louise flowing across a huge stage during a standing ovation from five thousand people—mostly women—who obviously adored her. Tall, slim, and elegant, as she walked to the podium I honestly felt that I could see a halo of goodness radiating from her blond bob. She arrived at the speaker's podium, but then, to let us know that she loved us and that she didn't want anything to come between us, she stepped out from behind the podium. She leaned against it casually and spoke to us in an ordinary voice, not as if she were giving a speech, but more intimately, as if we were all her best friends. I don't usually go for talk about the inner child, but she was so down-to-earth about it that it just seemed sensible to admit that there might be a baby inside us that needed befriending.

"She's an angel," I whispered to David and to my surprise, he nodded, also happily under her unique spell.

The next day I found out that modern-day saints are like the rest of us, especially if they are eighty-five years old. Exactly the same age as my mother, Louise had no time to waste and certainly wasn't going to spend the time she did have talking about theories when there was serious work to be done. Her secretary had managed to squeeze me into Louise's busy schedule, and at ten A.M. sharp I rang the bell on her hotel room door, surprised when Louise herself answered. She boomed, "Come on in! Have a seat while I clean up this table from last night."

She started clearing wineglasses off the round dining table as I walked over to the living room and plopped down in a corner of the couch. She joined me a moment later, looking fresh and vibrant and loose, sitting both with good posture and an easy slouch that reminded me she had once been a model. To suck up to her, I was wearing my favorite Japanese T-shirt, the cute one with the big pink fuzzy smiley face, that I hoped would immediately demonstrate that I was a deeply positive person. But right then what I actually felt was super nervous and even more so, since she was clearly super relaxed.

As I had suspected, she didn't have a clue who I was or what I was doing in her hotel living room or what she was supposed to do with me. So I got the ball rolling by introducing myself, reminding her of our mutual connections and how I came to be sitting there.

She listened to my spiel—"an epidemic of women hating their bodies . . . always wanting to be and look different . . . destroying so many women's self-confidence . . . I'm on a quest to find out how I can be of help and blah blah blah"—but she didn't seem to get hooked by my pitch the way Jamie Lee Curtis or Christiane Northrup had been.

In fact, there was already starting to be some dead air in this meeting. Being with Louise was like being with a vacuum cleaner that was sucking up my already minimal confidence and leaving me hanging out in space to dry. I rushed to fill in the gap by mentioning that this interview was in the service of a book I was writing called *I Hate My Body*.

That elicited a grunt from her. "Oh. Well. A lot of people say that and think that."

"Yes, a lot of people say that and think that, and it's a huge topic. I'm clearly not the first person to tackle it, but it's not really going away." I was already overly impassioned, trying to cook up enough energy for both of us because she wasn't biting.

She said, "Uh-huh."

"So . . . I'm talking to some people that I admire and that I think have a lot of insight, like you."

I was trying the buttering-up approach, but she was immune to that. She made no comment. Maybe I needed to tell her more about myself.

"I'm actually a pretty well-known yoga teacher all over the world. I have people looking at me as a role model and yet I feel a little like a fraud because—"

She interrupted me with a chuckle. "Oh, we all do! You know we have this idea that we have to be perfect if we teach, but if we could just realize that we only attract people to us that we can help. You know, you can't do the whole world. You can't!"

Then she sat up a bit as if agreeing to apply herself to the topic at hand. "I decided a long time ago I would make peace with my body. This is a progression that we all make—we come from a little fat baby and, if we make it, we go to one hundred. And we're meant to experience it all."

She continued. "I've noticed that just within the last three months I've gone into another shift of aging in my body. On one level I say to myself that it's sad, and on another level I go back to 'Louise, you've got to make peace with this. You feel good. You've got good energy. You take care of yourself.'"

I liked that. "So what you're saying is that making peace with your body is not something that happens once and for all and then you're done with it."

"It happens continually." She pointed to the skin on her arms. "Now the wrinkles are here. I've had these for a while, so I no longer wear certain things." Then she pointed to her stomach. "And I noticed just two or three weeks ago that now wrinkles are here, and there's really not much you can do about it," she said matter-of-factly.

Hearing Louise talking about this made a lightbulb go on for me. I had learned in my yoga practice that there are some smooth days and some rough days, but practicing yoga is never something that you give up on. Neither is it something that you master. The whole point is that you maintain commitment to the process, stay open to the changes that arise and pass, and most important, always take a friendly approach to your experience on the mat. This seemed to be the same process that Louise applied to how she related to her own body.

But she didn't want to dwell on the signs of aging in her body. I understood that she was teaching me something with that message, too: Not dwelling is an important part of the solution. As I was digesting this insight, she moved on to a larger view of her teaching:

"Whether we're happy or not is up to us. It has nothing to do with anybody else. It's the thoughts we choose to think and the foods we choose to eat that create healthy bodies."

I confessed, "I would never be mean to anybody else the way that I'm mean to myself."

Impatient with me, she barked, "So, what's so bad about you, anyway?"

This question stopped my mind. Louise Hay was the first woman I'd ever met who didn't say, "Yes, I know exactly what you mean, and I hate my body, too." She could say, "I'm working on feeling good about my aging body," but she wasn't going to give me an ounce of support for my drama. And she didn't particularly need to be sweet and sensitive about it either.

At a loss, I muttered, "Um, right. Actually there's nothing so bad about me and in fact, I think I deserve better from myself."

"But if you keep doing it, you will get more lines in your face!" She roared with uncontained laughter at that little dig. She'd caught me in her trap and she was having a ball! I was starting to understand that this was not an interview. This was surgery and she was a master of her craft. Louise was going to do whatever it took to get me to change my script, and she didn't mind if things got a little bit bloody.

She cut to the chase. "Do the people in your life love you?"

Without hesitation I responded, "Yes, they love me. And I've even been noticing lately, as I teach yoga all over the world, that even though I think I have a terrible body, I can feel how much the students love me. They don't care what my body looks like because they actually like me."

Louise just sat there looking at me, her shit detector on high alert. She was waiting for me to stop with the Sally Field act and tell her something real.

Then I surprised myself by saying, "Well, I would like to feel more love from my husband."

She jumped on this. "But you keep telling him what's wrong with you all the time. And he's tired of hearing it."

"Yeah, he's sick of it."

"So why do you do it?"

"I don't know. Why do I do it?"

"Beats me. Because you haven't forgiven. Who do you need to forgive? How did you learn to hate your body? Did your parents hate your body? Did they tell you to hate your body?"

"My mother was always on a diet. I think she hated her body."

"Okay! So you wanted to be a good girl like Mommy . . . and maybe her mother . . . ?"

"Her mother. I don't remember her that well, but she was always dressed . . ."

She knew the answer better than I did. "Perfectly?"

I nodded.

"Everybody had to be perfect."

I thought about this for a moment. "Maybe it is about flawlessness. My mother was a minister's wife. That means you can't be sexy. It's a good girl thing where your appearance has to be very clean and exactly right and then you'll be acceptable. So I still want that, I still want to look good."

"But, you see . . ." Louise shifted a bit and paused briefly. It seemed that this was all so obvious to her and that she had probably had this conversation a million times before. But she was willing to do it once more, so she leaned over to give me this news flash. "You've got to love the little kid inside . . . and you don't." Oh, I see, that inner child she was talking about yesterday meant me.

She softened her tone. "You've got to be willing to start trying."

"How do I do that?"

"Well, by changing the messages in your head. You're doing rotten affirmations. Nonstop."

She got personal again. "What would you like your relationship with your body to be like? You are not going backward, you are not going to have an eighteen-year-old body, so what would you like your relationship with your body to be like now?"

"More free, more friendly."

"What does that mean?"

"I feel like I have an addiction to hating my body and I'd like to be free of it."

"But I see a person sitting here who is not willing to make any changes."

"Well, I guess I'm talking about it but I'm not willing to . . ."

"You're talking about it but you're not DOING ANYTHING except irritating your husband!"

I responded meekly, "Yes, thank you for saying that. I'll think about it that way."

"You should! It's a pain in the ass to have somebody whining all the time about something they won't do anything about."

Louise might have been tough loving me but she wasn't ready to give up on me. She tried another angle. "Think of yourself as a new little yoga student. Because I feel you're gentle with your students."

How did she know that? It made me feel good that she saw that in me. Her method seemed to be that she cracked you open like an egg, separating the protein-rich white stuff from vitamin-heavy yolk so she could see what was rotten and then gently reintegrate all that gooey stuff into a stronger whole. She knew that you don't have to be a perfect circle to be a good egg.

I softened, thinking of all the yogis in my classes. "Oh, with my students, I'm so . . ."

Louise turned a huge smile on me because she knew where this was going.

". . . kind. So much kinder to them, you know. . . ."

She did know. She knew I meant kinder to them than to myself. She encouraged me to go on. "Yes, yes."

"I love them and I don't care what they look like and I never think their bodies are wrong or anything like that."

"And you see them become more beautiful."

"Yes, and more confident. And it makes me feel great."

Louise was chuckling, pleased with this little breakthrough. Now she was ready to let me go. We stood up together. "You're looking younger than when you walked in. Wrinkles fade when tensions dissipate. They can do that very quickly."

She stood facing me. "I want you to say to yourself a lot: *I am my own yoga student.*"

"I am my own yoga student," I repeated.

"And . . . when you interview other people, don't tell them how much you hate your body. Stop that. Just stop it. You can say this is a problem I used to have and I'm really working on it and I'm going to help other women. But don't say"—and here she whispered because she didn't want to say it herself—"'I hate my body,' because every time you say it, it just gets . . . worse."

She looked me in the eye to elicit my agreement. "So we're not going to say that anymore. If you do say it, then put it in the past tense. Because when you get it, you're going to get it for everybody."

I sighed. "Well, that's my hope."

"No, no. That's what you know. That's what you're doing. You are in the process of doing that. Call me if you need a boost up." She grabbed a pen. "Let me give you my number. Once you are on the path, you know a sentence or two can mean a lot."

"That's what I was wondering about. What happens when you backslide?"

"Don't worry about that. The process of doing affirmations or doing any of these things is you practice, you forget. You practice, you forget. That's when a lot of people go, 'Ahhhh, you see, I can't do it right, I can't do it right.' No, you practice and you forget and then you catch yourself. That's to be celebrated. You know how it is when you watch a yoga student and they get into the posture and it's wrong and then they make a self-adjustment. That's when you think . . ."

I jumped in: "Oh good—they're getting it!"

"Yes, and the student herself may be thinking, 'Oh God, I'm wrong again,' but she self-adjusted. Well, that's what you need to do with affirmations—just self-adjust. You're not going to go into every posture perfectly and have it perfect forever and ever and ever."

She smiled at me. "Isn't it interesting how we don't see things that are right here? Right here."

We walked to the door together and she gave me a final send-off. "So, be kind to this new student. You've got a new student, and new students often walk in a little shaky. And, one of those times when you get stuck, give me a call. You are entering a new posture."

She gave me a big hug and I walked out the door back to the elevator, down ten floors and into our room where David was sitting on the bed with his computer. "Well, how did it go?" he asked. And I burst into tears.

It was Valentine's Day, and I was out of town. I had brought my mom a dozen roses the day before I left the city. Though I didn't like to admit it, she wouldn't have known what day it was anyway. I cut the stems short and put the flowers in a small rose-colored ceramic vase. "Mom, I brought you some roses," I said, holding them under her nose.

I rarely saw her with her eyes open these days. Tubby, the head nurse, told me that sometimes Millie did open her eyes, just not when I came to visit. "You put her right to sleep," she teased me. "That happens with mothers and daughters." Tubby had a theory that the moms felt safe when their daughters were there, so they closed their eyes and relaxed. I didn't know. I thought that my mom's brain just worked in a different way. Her vivid dreamscape held her attention more easily than the sights and sounds of the world that I was living in.

Twenty years ago, just before my mom's sixty-fifth birthday, she and I had gone shopping at the Farmers Market in Dallas. We saw a display of pottery and a little card advertising classes. When she said, "I think I'd like to try that," I got my dad to go in halves with me and we bought her a six-week session for her birthday present. She was hooked by the second class. Making pottery became my mom's passion and one of the great joys of her life. Never mind that she turned out to be exceptionally talented, winning blue ribbons at the annual Dallas Craft Fair; she just loved doing it. I think it had a lot to do with the tactile aspect, handling the clay and shaping it into something beautiful and useful, the same way she had done with fabric when I was growing up.

Now my house is full of those memories: Leroy's water dish with the painting of a puppy who has ears more like a cat's than a poodle's; the elegant footed fruit bowl on my dining room table; the pink handle-less mug that holds my drawing pencils; the tiny vases that hold one small blossom each.

I thought she might like to have one of her own vases in her room at the nursing home. She didn't feel like opening her eyes the day I brought it to her so I placed her hand on the little rose-colored vase. Maybe she would recognize the double ridge she'd carved just below the narrow opening. She did! The minute she felt her vase she smiled and it was clear that she knew what she was touching.

The feeling for the clay was still in her fingers, even though she couldn't do anything with her hands anymore. Up until a few months ago she would repetitively open and close her fingers, balling up the covers of her bed or the front of her shirt. Then she'd say, "Could you hold this for me?" I'd slide the fabric out of her hand, saying, "Sure, Mom. I've got it now." Then she would relax. A second or two later, she would do it all again. But now she was too weak to even do that gesture, and so her ladylike hands stayed in her lap, fingers curled in, a constant tremor in both wrists.

There was something familiar about those hands in that lap. I recognized the quiet gracefulness, yes, and also the recessed aspect of my mom, too—a deep sense of privacy and shyness. Maybe I shouldn't have been surprised that her interior life was more compelling than the reality of life in a nursing home. She was never great at engaging in any potentially uncomfortable exchange.

When it was time to teach me about the birds and the bees, she picked me up from school, took me home, handed me a pamphlet, and told me to read it. If I had any questions afterward, I could ask her. I felt total embarrassment, as in "dying of." I stormed into the living room, plopped down on the couch, and skimmed the pamphlet on menstruation. God, do we really have to do this, Mom?

Now, of course, I realize that she was embarrassed, too, or she would have done the whole thing differently. But her impersonal approach also made me mad. I read the book in ten minutes and went to find my mom, who was primping in the bathroom, getting ready to go out with my dad. I glared at her as she worked on her hair.

"Did you finish?" She didn't put her curling iron down.

"Yeah, and I already know all that stuff anyway."

"Okay."

End of story. Almost. She pulled open the drawer where she kept her fat pile of sanitary napkins. "Here's the Kotex and a belt for you. Do you know how to use it?"

I didn't really but, ewww, it was all so icky and awkward. "Yes," I said in a snotty voice and stormed off to the living room.

A few years later I asked my mom if I could switch to tampons. It took me months to get up the nerve to even bring up the subject. As I expected, she resisted at first, and then very begrudgingly allowed it. I could feel that she thought there was something not quite "good girl" about tampons, maybe something sexual. I realize now she didn't want me to be all that familiar with my vagina or the feeling of anything going in and out of there. I sensed something about her attitude, which made me feel slightly dirty. But I wasn't a slut. I just knew that all my friends were using tampons and it was way better than having that lumpy thing sticking out between your legs, making the back of your skirt ride up in a way that let everyone know—including boys—that you were having your period.

Is it possible that I might have been more sexually confident if my mom hadn't passed on her embarrassment to me? It is possible that I would have felt altogether different about my body? It wasn't until many years after adolescence when I moved to New York and met a new friend, a lovely Wicca woman, who mentioned that she was having her "pyramid," that I got a new perspective on what Christiane Northrup calls our "power spots."

In the hallway, I grabbed Dr. Griffo, who had been treating my mom's acute bedsore, for an update on her condition. He smiled a New Yorker's kind of sideways smile. "Pardon me for saying so, but well, there isn't really anything wrong with your mom from the neck down, if you know what I mean. Her vital signs are excellent, and she is not dying." Within three weeks at the skilled nursing facility, her mind started to break down.

The home was full of people whose bodies and minds were on parallel but separate tracks. Maureen's other client, also in her late eighties, broke her ankle and right away her mind just went. Chicken and egg was unclear to me, but there was no doubt that mind and body are intricately connected. Dr. Griffo wanted to put my mom back on a physical-therapy program now that her bedsore had started healing up, but he said she had to be willing to open her eyes.

So I held the roses under her nose. "Mmm, don't they smell

good, Mom?" No response. She was dissolving. She looked peaceful, though, and I thought how happy she would be if she knew that she finally lost those fifty pounds.

———◆———

It was quiet when I walked to the yoga studio in Shibuya on Monday morning. I thought maybe I'd gotten my days mixed up—that can happen with jet lag. There simply weren't enough people at the station crosswalk for it to be a Monday morning. The multidirectional Shibuya crossing is called the Scramble and it typically takes about five light changes and ten minutes to get across. I had been trained by my Japanese yoga friends to point myself straight ahead and when the light turns green, just go—never swerve or even look sideways, or the crowds will devour you. Today the Scramble was empty.

It was March 14, a cold, gray day with no hint of spring in the air. I hadn't fully grokked that the power outages in Tokyo were keeping so many people home, even preventing some of the big chain stores from opening. I just knew something was off and I felt unsettled and low, as if the cold-and-gray-ness was coming from inside me.

I was in Japan to teach the second annual OM yoga Teacher Training course here, hosted by TokyoYoga. This was my fourth teaching trip to Japan and I'd been looking forward to it. I love the culture—the graceful way money is exchanged on small trays; the taxi driver's white gloves and the lace doily cab-seat covers; the elegance of everyday bowing rituals; the shoes-off-inside policy; the deep respect for teachers; and the dinner custom I was taught in which one must never pour one's own drink but must always wait for your friends to fill and refill your sake cup.

In fact, only three days earlier I had been admiring the refined manners of the immigration officer in Narita airport. I liked how he took each new visitor's passport with both hands and returned it with a bow. As I watched him do that, I stood up straighter, gearing up my own mindfulness practice so that I could meet him with equal grace. But when I handed him my passport he turned his head and became very still. "That's weird." I got paranoid. "Is he trying to psych me out?" In the eyeblink moment it took to have that thought, I realized the officer was listening to something with his whole body.

Boom! I crumpled onto the edge of the luggage counter and felt an inner panic as the floor buckled and the overhead lamps started swinging. The room was suddenly noisy, full of wild grumblings in surround sound and violent pitching like airplane turbulence.

Long seconds later, as the whole thing just got bigger, I tried to comfort myself. "This must be the peak of it." That's when a ceiling panel fell down followed by a cascade of dust and the officer pointed to the swaying lights. Yes, I see, I should stand with the other people over by the baggage-claim area.

No one said a word. Passengers and officers and airport workers were all stunned into silence. I can't say I was shocked to experience an earthquake in Japan. Last year while teaching in Shinjuku, in mid-vinyasa, all the students dropped to the floor. They called, "Shyndi, Shyndi, earthquake!" And down I went, too. My reaction time to feeling an earthquake was slower than my Japanese students', just like it was with the immigration officer's.

Finally, the rumbling stopped. I don't remember it slowing down, just at one point the quiet included the environment, not just the people. I didn't hear any more creaking metal or what sounded like a truck driving through the wall. A completely compelling 3-D event had come and gone, just like that. The officers unfroze and looked at one another, seeming to communicate although I couldn't hear them say anything. A few stepped out of the room and a few others stepped into the room. Minutes passed, and then the immigration officer looked at me, nodding to indicate that I could return to the counter to retrieve my passport. I like to imagine that, even after having just experienced the biggest earthquake in recorded history, we still managed to exchange a final elegant bow but honestly, I don't remember. I just know I felt shaky and unstable, but I pulled it together and walked out the door.

I figured I'd do what I always do when I arrive in Japan: exchange money and then cross the hall to buy a bus ticket to my hotel. There were already people lined up at the currency exchange table and it seemed all was proceeding as normal. Okay, I get it—impermanence. Things are one way and then they are a different way, and people in Japan are used to earthquakes. Yen in hand, it was time to buy a bus ticket.

Boom! The earthquake was back, almost as agitated as before. Two Japanese women in pink bows and knee socks dropped to the floor next to me. Cries and shrieking all around. No more business as usual. This much moving force so soon after the first can't be taken in stride.

When the bucking slowed down, an announcement was made in Japanese. From the response I guessed it said, "Nobody move." In this culture based on obedience and respect, people simply complied, putting themselves on hold. But for me—all this shaking and rocking and plummeting to the floor and no one to talk to—it was just too isolating. So I did what any true New Yorker would do. I leaned over to a blond guy in a red shirt and tortoise-shell glasses and asked, "So . . . what do you think is going on?" He turned an open face to me and said, "I have no idea but it seems like they want us to go out into the parking lot where there isn't anything overhead that could fall on us." Out we went.

Brad and I stuck together in the parking lot. At first we tried to figure out what was going on but when even the official-looking types didn't have any answers, we just relaxed into the situation. We talked about why we were in Japan and where we came from and how we wished the announcements would be in English sometimes. What else could we do?

Two hours, three hours passed. We took each other's pictures on our cell phones. I couldn't get a Wi-Fi connection to email my picture to David but at least it would make a good Facebook post when I got to Tokyo. It was weird having no idea when that might be but at least having someone to talk with gave me a sense of grounding in that completely ungrounded situation.

If this had been a movie, the sky would have been dark, with sullen, threatening overtones. Instead the day was crisp and sunny, a refreshing almost-spring day, sending a confusing message of welcome. The weather seemed out of sync with the events of the day: sleep deprivation, jet lag, and terra non-firma.

By six P.M. the temperature had cooled off enough for us to really want to be back inside. We pulled our jackets tighter. Half an hour later, the crowd started moving back into the airport. I hadn't felt any more aftershocks and assumed that we would be able to get on the bus soon. But who knew? We sheep were simply herded back inside, where I found myself standing beneath the arrivals/departures board, which declared the status of all flights as indefinite. "Got any news?" I butted my nose into another guy's business when I saw him checking his BlackBerry. He said, "Eight-point-nine, off the northeast coast and there was a tsunami, too."

That was Joe and he'd made friends with Maya and Gary. In one instant, we became a group of five. Maya is Japanese so she told us what the announcements said, which was nothing much. Gary, an American IT expert living in Tokyo with his family, shared his impressions of how the Japanese deal with emergency situations. He told us they aren't facile with on-the-spot or out-of-the-box thinking. Clearly it was going to take a while for authorities to make a plan B and in the meantime, we were told that the trains weren't running and neither were the buses, since the entire highway was now closed. Japanese caution seemed to require that everything would be closed down until everything could be opened up.

That included the airport restaurants and stores. Along with eight thousand other people and no food or drink, we understood we would be spending the night in Narita. We claimed our territory under a backlit poster of Mount Fuji and set up camp. We heard a rumor that sleeping bags were being provided, so Joe and I volunteered to wait in the long line, nearly the full length of the airport. Joe, a retired vice admiral in the U.S. Coast Guard, with tons of experience in rescue missions, was a good person to be with, calm and patient in an emergency. Forty-five minutes later, when we were about twenty people from the front of the line, we were told, with much bowing and apologizing, that there were no more sleeping bags. There were no more Ritz crackers, either, but we did score some bottles of water.

In the meantime, Maya found a vending machine, one of the complicated Japanese ones that I can never figure out, and managed to buy us some hot drinks: "cohee," milk "cohee," and cocoa. Brad approached some people with extra sleeping bags and between his Midwestern friendliness and the unwavering Japanese good manners, he was able to get one for each of us. It was midnight by now and very cold.

The phone lines were jammed and I still couldn't get my email up and running. We all wanted to let our friends and family know we were okay but for now, we settled in. Gary pulled a few cords and other gadgets out of his pack and went to work getting online.

Sleeping wasn't really an option and we ended up sitting on the floor with our legs crossed like yogis while we shared our stories. It surprised my earthquake buddies to learn that I taught yoga all over the world. "Oh great! Can you show us some stretches?" Maya asked. That made me laugh but I was glad that I, too, could contribute something to the well-being of our group. Maya followed along as I did some twists and side bends, which felt good, but everybody's hips were starting to ache from the cold, hard floor and I knew I wasn't the only one who felt toxified from the whole situation, stressed out from the unknown.

That's where my earthquake friends came in. Maybe we were all in shock but not one of us complained even once. People tell me now that I was brave, but it wasn't like that. After those first big quakes, I never felt as if I were in immediate danger. It wasn't until later that I learned of the tremendous destruction resulting from the Pacific Rim rattling its bones and shifting the earth on its axis.

———◆·———

Twelve hours after we'd gone inside from the parking lot, I was back out there waiting for a taxi. At six A.M. on Saturday morning, I picked my way through sleeping bodies to the train station ticket counter, where a Japanese woman, still looking perfect in her uniform—accessorized with bandana and pillbox hat—kept repeating, "Yes, please. Train later." We knew the roads were still closed so buses were not an option either.

I assumed there would be huge lines of waiting taxis and waiting taxi passengers, just as there would be if this were Newark Liberty Airport. But there were only ten people and zero taxis. It was cold, but I was determined. Every twenty minutes a lone taxi showed up. The taxi dispatcher said the highway to Tokyo was still closed, but we could get a ride to Chiba, an hour-and-a-half ride.

Chiba? Where is Chiba? Hoo, boy. Fortunately, Hiro was

also waiting for a taxi and offered to help me get there. When we exited the taxi in Chiba, Hiro simply picked up my extra-large suitcase and went, me scurrying after him, pushing through the crowds to the one local train that was running toward Tokyo. Another train, several subways and a short walk through Shibuya—Hiro carrying my suitcase for the entire six-and-a-half hours—and he delivered me to the front desk of the Cerulean Tower Hotel with a deep bow. He still had another hour of travel to get to his home, but his generosity dictated he take care of me first. In these kinds of situations you meet some angels and some devils.

The Cerulean was party central. The dire consequences of the earthquake were still unknown so, at that point, being stuck in Japan became an unexpected holiday. The massive lobby was heavily populated with groovy people wearing the international groovy people's uniform: jeans, T-shirts with a geeky phrase like LONDON ROCKS! that is really insider lingo for "I'm a hipster jet-setter"; brightly colored sneakers; porkpies or Yankees caps; necks wrapped with gingham. I relaxed back into civilization and started to feel safe again.

After I settled into my room on the thirty-third floor, I rang up my husband over iChat, grateful that Gary had finally man-aged to send an email to him the night before. Frantic about my safety, his big face loomed into the screen. "Have you seen the news? Do you really know what's going on over there?"

"Well, yeah, David, sure I do. I'm the one who was actually in the earthquake." I explained to him that what he was seeing on the news was hundreds of miles away and things in Tokyo were normal. The teacher training was going to go on as planned. After the cold, hard floor of the airport, I was ecstatic to be in my fancy hotel room and couldn't wait to get into my cushy hotel bed. I calmed him down and then slept for nine hours straight.

———— • ◆ • ————

The next day the training started and although two people were absent because of travel complications from the earthquake, I was able to lead the first day of yoga classes with a reasonable amount of ease. That morning while I was checking my email, I felt a couple of aftershocks, which unnerved me. I had a startled response each time the heat kicked on in my room, and when the plastic of my Perrier bottle popped, I nearly jumped out of my skin. I hurried through necessary things such as sitting on the toilet and taking a shower, not places I wanted to be if another big earthquake happened.

But I wasn't nervous at all while I was teaching. Even though it's my time to teach and not to "do" yoga, my own clear instructions and soothing voice affected me in a similar way as they did my students, and I experienced a kind of yoga contact high. As a result I felt balanced, openhearted, and confident as I walked back to the hotel. I passed a line of about a hundred nervous people waiting for the bus, clutching their bags and holding their arms tight to their chests, standing in silence across from a dimmed Shibuya Station, normally the most riotous wall of light and sound in Tokyo. That gave me a contact low.

Alone after a day of teaching and not yet hungry enough for dinner, I sat down at my computer and once again felt woozy—did I just feel another earthquake or was that my imagination? Feeling the motion of an earthquake even when there isn't one is called *jishin yoi,* which means "earthquake drunk." I didn't know that one of the ways to treat it is to lie down, but that's what I did. I got down on the floor, the closest I could get to the earth, and did what I do whenever I want to be home—I rolled out my mat.

———— ✦ ————

Downward Dog is a magic pill. Pushing down with hands and heels feels grounding and turns my organs upside down, giving my heart a healthy massage.

If I had known about the radiation meltdowns, I might have hesitated to breathe so deeply and fully, but so far I only knew about the earth and the water. Finding a point on the wall to help me balance, I practice Tree Pose and Half Moon Pose and don't feel wobbly at all. Training one's eyes on a distant object is also a remedy for being earthquake drunk.

Down on my back, I scooch around, ending up on a diagonal, feet near the end of the bed, arms overhead in the space between the bedside table and the desk. From here I can lift one leg straight up to the ceiling and take it across my body into a nourishing spinal twist and hip releaser.

It is good to be back in my body, focused on my breath, reintegrated through the refuge of my practice. *Yoga* means "union," but really, it's reunion. We disintegrate all the time; it doesn't take an earthquake for that to happen. A hundred times a day we notice that our mind and body are living in different realms of space and time, but that's no problem. Yoga, like meditation, offers a method for coming together after you've come apart.

That day Japan was still shaking its skeleton while the massive tsunami pools were hardening into ice. Soon enough we would learn that the fires burning in the nuclear reactors were tainting the seawater and the air; bad winds were blowing south toward Tokyo. I knew that nothing is solid, everything is impermanent, everything is meant to change. But I tried not to think about any of that. I tried to keep my mind and my body in one place, the safe harbor I was creating in the five feet between my bed and the window, where I was afraid to look out because it seemed so far to the ground.

My practice ends, as always, with a headstand and shoulder stand followed by Savasana, a resting pose lying flat on my back. Finally, rolling over to one side, I let my head dangle as I round up through every single vertebra, settling into Sukhasana. I fold my hands the way Rimpoche taught me, fingertips touching with thumbs tucked into the palms.

All day I'd been fighting an intense longing to go home. But I feel better now, less scared. The feeling in my bones and muscles, lungs and belly reminds me that yoga is my home. It is a place I can always return to.

My practice always concludes by dedicating the benefits of my practice to all beings everywhere, but that day I aim my wishes for compassion, freedom from suffering, joy, and equanimity directly to the people of Japan.

———— ◆ ————

While getting dressed for the second day of teacher training, I tried to watch CNN, but in contrast to the quiet void-like vibe of Tokyo, Anderson Cooper seemed hysterical, although he wasn't yet wearing his disaster hoodie. I turned off the TV and left for the studio, crossing the empty Scramble without even stopping at the curb.

Already informed that even more students would miss today's session due to power outages that had caused subway cancellations, I was asked to end the day early so those who were there could catch a train before dark. We decided to cut the lunch break short, which was fine by me. I never know what to do on my lunch break in Japan anyway, because I can't read most menus, and my host always tries to send me to the local, smoke-filled Denny's; perhaps he is under the impression that I will be comfortable with the familiar menu but Denny's typical un-yogic fare of French fries is not what I want to eat in America and certainly not in Japan.

I decided to go to Seibu, a big department store that had just opened a new "food show" floor, where I thought I might be able to get something to eat that wasn't completely mysterious to me. Just because I was spending my lunch hour in a store, I told myself I wasn't really shopping, which somehow felt unseemly in the midst of a disastrous time. I might just browse a bit and check out what was "in" in Japan this season.

Good intentions aside, I soon found myself asking to try on a pair of red gingham Spanish espadrilles, which I happened to know you cannot buy anywhere in NYC. The escalator up to the restaurant passed several Japanese designer's in-store boutiques, where I was once again magnetized to those bias-cut, baggy pants and blousey smock tops that are perfect on the typical waif-like Japanese woman. Nothing will look good on big old American me, I reminded myself. Even the espadrilles were too tight, my big toe gushing out of the pointy-toe peephole, the heel straps instantly giving me a blister. The shoe lady told me they don't even carry size eights in that store.

After partially finishing a weird salad involving mysterious tentacle-like ingredients that I didn't recognize and avoided eating, I left Seibu feeling diminished by the whole experience. It wasn't just the overcast day or lack of the normal upbeat urban energy. I felt fat . . . again. It didn't matter that I hadn't eaten much. Being jet-lagged makes me bloated and gives me an excuse to visit my go-to place, which is "the land of I'm fat." For me, feeling fat is not necessarily a physical feeling. I can feel fat even when I haven't eaten anything. Feeling fat is actually my mental comfort zone; a little round bed for my grumpy voice to become full throated and tell me once again that I was fat . . . and old . . . and hopeless. To berate myself for being here again, back in Japan, traveling too much to ever get on a roll with my exercise program or consistent with a healthy diet and anyway . . .

I stopped at the crosswalk and joined the good citizens of Tokyo, who waited patiently for the long red light to finally turn green. Feeling chilly, I tightened the scarf around my neck and stared into space. I settled down a little bit and got bored. And as I waited, I relaxed. I thought about something and then I thought about nothing. Some space in my mind opened up in a natural way.

Then a new thought popped up. "Oh, my habit is really coming on strong today. That's interesting."

Ding! In that moment, I woke up out of my fog and saw that this whole thing, the whole I-Hate-My-Body drama, was something outside of me. For the first time, it wasn't me and it wasn't a truth. It was just a thing that sometimes comes up, like when I noticed that my hips were tight from sitting at my desk all day or my shoulders were sore from yoga. It was part of me, but not all of me. And it was only part of me for a little while and then it changed and went away. Just like my tight hips got loosened up with some stretching, this thought was not permanent or solid or even true.

For so many years I had been doing everything it took to strengthen the belief that my body was not good enough, which meant that I'm not good enough, which meant I needed to change something, do more, be different, take some action. I felt sure that if only I could figure out the right doing, the precise corrective, I'd finally have a good body and then I'd be happy. Just like doing reps with weights, I had exercised this neural pathway so many times that it had developed into a firm and muscle-bound point of view.

But in the past few years, this pattern had become more apparent to me as a self-imposed form of torture, which I was consciously working to dismantle. I guess that I had been working on stretching it long enough—turning it upside down, wondering how it started, trying to locate its power, pushing it away, tipping it off center—and it was finally loosened up and losing its hold on me.

Was it being in an earthquake that shook it all loose? Or perhaps it was the sense of loss and upset in my marriage that helped me see the holes in my ossified logic. Like a mini-satori, the Zen-like thunderbolt of sudden awareness, I thought, "Oh yeah, I recognize you. You're that kind of thinking that always comes up when I'm feeling low."

In the past, I would have responded to that thought with self-destructive strategies like shopping—even if the stores didn't carry my size—or eating and drinking too much. In fact, wasn't I just trying on too small espadrilles and longing for a skinny Japanese body so I could wear those baggy pants? But at this moment, I simply didn't respond. Like an advanced yoga student, I heard the words but I stayed steady and rested, using the gap to give myself a chance to find out what was really going on.

Just like puzzling out the source of a bad feeling in my stomach, it was the familiar feeling of the negative thought that caught my attention. What was really bothering me? As the tide of habit ebbed, I realized that I was very anxious about the situation in Tokyo. I thought, "Give yourself a break. You've just been in a bunch of very big earthquakes. You are in a foreign country where you don't know the language, and the country is in a crisis. You are alone and it's cold outside. No wonder you are feeling out of sorts. You need to find someone who can help you."

I had been stuck, and now I was unstuck. I didn't know what to do next but I felt stronger than my habit in a way that was liberating and put a fire under my ass.

As soon as I got back to the studio, I asked my translator Yukiko to let me talk to John, her Canadian husband. She rolled her eyes as she auto-dialed his number, telling the other yogis that he was going to scare me. She was right. John told me that things were only going to get worse. "There's already no bread on the shelves, and who knows what's going to happen next. The Canadian and U.S. embassies are recommending all citizens return home." John had already left Tokyo and taken their children to Osaka, where he said the hotel was full of ex-pats concerned about lack of food, gas shortages, and radiation poisoning. I thanked him profusely, went back to my hotel, and booked a flight for Newark.

It was the 6.4 that struck while I was having dinner with my hosts that evening in a fourteenth-floor restaurant that finally did me in. My host had just finished expressing his appreciation for how well I handled the students that afternoon. "You were so professional," he said with a small bow. We made a toast but after only one sip of sake I felt swoony. Embarrassed, I thought, "My gosh, am I so fried that I'm drunk on one sip of sake?" It was another big earthquake, and then another one struck ten minutes later. That was it for me. My nerves were shot. There was no way I could handle another night on a high floor, swaying through more aftershocks.

When I got back to my deserted hotel at midnight, the fun vibe had morphed into a palpable sense of foreboding. The vaulted lobby was empty, every restaurant closed, hotel workers in their uniforms waiting to be helpful, but there was literally not one person but me to help. There was one taxi in the driveway and I nabbed it. Seventy-five minutes and four-hundred dollars later, my driver bowed and left me on the curb. Five nights after I arrived in Japan I was back at the airport. The entire first night I'd spent at Narita the fluorescents remained on, but now with the imposed power outages, it was quiet and dark.

I was nervous and wondered if the airport was even open, but I saw a few people schlepping bags, so I followed them, hoping they knew where the door was, because I sure didn't. The hotel receptionist had cautioned me, "There will be a lot of people at the airport tonight. Please be careful."

As I stepped inside the dim entryway of the departure terminal, I saw a security guard on patrol. I figured after I made a pit stop I'd settle in for the night, so I asked him directions to the ladies'. Like Hiro, he didn't just point but politely escorted me all the way to the door of the bathroom. When I came out, I didn't feel afraid, just a little bit lonely.

So I did what had worked before—I looked around to see if I could find someone who might speak my language. And guess what? There was Brad, sleeping on a bench right in front of me! I rolled my suitcase over and plopped down on the floor, prepared to wait through the night with my earthquake friend.

When I'd first told David my earthquake story he said, "Really? The minute you handed the guy your passport the earthquake hit? Wow, Cyndi, you're so powerful!" David wasn't kidding. From his vantage point—twenty-four hours a day in front of the TV—the hyper-agitation of CNN's reporting filled him with anxiety and perhaps a sense of the mythological.

To some, the massive earthquake and the constant aftershocks seemed like an urgent message from the earth. I read email conversations on CNN's website from viewers who argued that the cause of the earthquake was Japan's insistence on killing sharks for soup. Others replied that that's not how karma works; some wrote that there is no meaning to any of this and everybody should get a grip.

Before I left for Japan, David and I had been in the Cleveland airport and we stopped to watch a charming Rube Goldberg display. It was a brightly painted contraption made up of wire spirals, scales, ramps, ladders, and springs through which Ping-Pong balls traveled in various directions, depending on how or when the next ball arrived. The first ball didn't get pushed out of the tunnel until one, two, three, four, and then finally the fifth ball's force pushed it over the edge. From there it landed on a spring that bounced it to the top of a chute, down which it slid, landing on the bottom rung of a mechanical ladder that carried the ball back to the top to begin again. A visual example of interdependence, this motorized perpetual motion machine came to mind as the situation in Japan devolved further each day I was there. The earth shook, the water rose up, the power plants shut down, the electricity went off, the people dealt with it as best they could.

We'd been in Cleveland to teach our workshop on the Six Perfections—the actions of a bodhisattva—an almost Buddha with perfect compassion. But in Japan I found that nobody needed a teaching on generosity, discipline, patience, diligence, meditation, or wisdom. It was natural for people in Japan to take care of one another, control their minds, remain calm, maintain their stamina, stay focused, and make choices that would be good for everyone.

It had taken courage on my part to make a decision regarding the teacher training. Yesterday I took my teacher's seat, legs folded in Vajrasana, the Basic Goodness Pose, which is also called Hero's Pose. It means that the Hero is you, the person who sits quietly and openly, brave enough to face your own fears. I faced my Japanese students and took a moment to feel connected to my Basic Goodness. Then I expressed myself with honesty as I told them that I felt it was best to postpone the training. There were lots of tears from them but no bad vibes. When BG is on full display everyone feels it. Inspired by the nobility and elegance of the Japanese people, I managed to express graceful leadership in a manner that I hoped left the door open for my future return to TokyoYoga.

Sitting in the semidarkness of the airport, I felt as if I were on a threshold, a liminal space between now and then, known and unknown. I felt strong and oddly grounded, in a land where the ground is hyper-mobile. I felt good that I had figured out how to take care of myself in a very challenging situation, with minimal support and a lot of mixed messages.

I read that according to Shinto, the ancient religion of Japan, the invisible space of a doorway is what both separates and unites two opposite worlds. It is still everyday tradition for a visitor approaching someone's home to call out, "*Ojama shimasu.*" Used in the same way, we might say, "May I come in?" The literal translation is, "I am about to disturb you." I didn't know what my life would be like when I got back. It might be full of disturbances. But I was strangely confident that I could handle whatever I met upon my return.

David was so relieved that I was coming home early that he rented a car to pick me up at the airport. In seventeen years, he had never done that before. He also emailed that he was praying to the water and earth gods and dragons to protect me. I appreciated that, I really did.

But I liked it better when my earthquake friend, Joe, said,

"It's gonna take a while for those shifting plates to settle." No need for more drama, thank you. If I took it personally, there would be a feeling of malignancy, which led only to confusion, fear, anxiety, guilt—all kinds of stuff that wasn't really needed or useful or accurate. The earth moved. It does that sometimes. It was not about me.

As my Continental flight began its descent into Newark, the senior flight attendant finished her disembarkation announcements by saying, "From the beaches of Waikiki to the oranges of California, from the majesty of the Rocky Mountains to the Statue of Liberty, may I be the first to welcome you home to the golden arms of the USA. I am glad to have brought all two hundred seventy-eight of you home safely. Our prayers are with the brave people of Japan." Maybe that was corny, but it meant a lot to me, and when I looked around the cabin I saw that I wasn't the only one crying.

I'm down in a low squat, demonstrating how to help a yoga student use blocks in a forward bend. Jackie has been working hard on her yoga practice, but she still can't fold all the way forward without rounding her back and bending her knees. So I patiently explain that if she places her hands on blocks it will lift her spine, allowing her to straighten her legs. Then she can extend through her spine and start to feel the benefits of this wonderful pose.

We're in the middle of an OM yoga Teacher Training course, and the students are fascinated by these detailed explanations. They watch closely as I work with every student, and each time someone improves even incrementally, it feels like a victory for everyone. The class bursts into applause!

I say to Jackie, "If you keep working, you'll get where you want to go. You can't skip steps and hope to arrive magically at a full forward bend. But using blocks will help to lengthen your hamstrings and strengthen your back muscles and you will get there soon enough. And"—I pause to emphasize that I want to encourage her and acknowledge her hard work—"you've come a long way. Your pose is much more open than it was when you started practicing. You're doing great."

Jackie rolls up through her spine, arriving back in a standing position. She smiles and I can tell she really appreciates what I said. But I feel that she is holding something back.

I look at her. "Do you want to say something?"

With a rush, she confesses, "I think maybe my arms are just too short."

Everyone laughs, including Jackie.

I say, "Oh yes, let's blame it on the arms! I can guarantee you that in this class there is someone who has arms that are too long, or their legs are too short or too thick, or they are too old or too stiff or too tall or too loose or too tight . . ." The class is really laughing now.

"The thing is, Jackie, we are used to thinking yoga will change our body to the way we want it to be—taller, thinner, stronger, more fluid—and then, and only then, will we really be able to 'do' yoga. But we can only ever do yoga with the body we have in this very moment, right now.

"The first sutra or line of scripture from the traditional philosophy of yoga reads, 'Yoga is now.' It's a mandate to relate to yourself as you are. When we take our short arms and flabby thighs and gripped abdominals and bunions and muscle-bound shoulders, not to mention our bad mood and our burning ambition and our irritating, competitive nature—take all of that onto the mat with us and do yoga with all that in the mix—then we are doing yoga. And then if our arms get longer and our legs get thinner we won't care anymore. It's not about that. We will be integrated—my favorite definition of yoga.

"So, I'm sorry to break the news, but you can't blame anything on your arms. And what's more"—I pause again both for dramatic effect and because what I am about to say is the most important lesson of teacher training—"there's nothing wrong with you."

The class is suddenly still and quiet.

"There never has been and there never will be."

Jackie's face is open and a little bit pinky and flushed. I hold her eyes with mine. She doesn't cry, but I almost do.

———— ✦ ————

The couch in our West Village apartment molded to my body in a way that suggested I need never get up. Perfect. I accepted that invitation and curled into a ball where I stayed for hours, sobbing and cooking up more reasons to feel bad. I was having a total relapse from positive thinking. Just like any kind of recovery program, in which the addict makes progress and then finds herself back in a bar, smoking and drinking, I had lost faith in the possibility of lightness. My heart was heavy and so were my thoughts.

"Can I ever get a new boyfriend? Will anyone ever want me: a gray-haired, fifty-something with flab? No, everybody wants women twenty years younger than I am. No one will ever want me. My whole life is a mess. How did it happen that the promise of my young life became such a big, fat mess that all

I can do is lie in a puddle of sorrow on my couch in the middle of the afternoon?" Thinking this way made me cry more.

Back in my familiar surroundings, the awakening I'd experienced in Japan had dissolved but nothing had arisen in its place. Without another big trip or project to focus on, I had no choice but to hang out in the confusion of my life. I'd been trying to abide in a state of not knowing, as one of my meditation teachers once recommended. He also kindly said that doing so takes a lot of composure.

My original plan for that evening had not been to collapse in a heap and become immobile. In fact, I'd really been looking forward to going to the Shambhala Meditation Center to see Jetsunma Tenzin Palmo. Jetsunma was an inspiration to me and many others for her profound commitment to becoming enlightened in a female body. After being on retreat in a Himalayan cave for twelve years, she now traveled around the world giving teachings in order to raise funds for the nunnery she founded to educate Indian girls.

Years before, I'd met her at a private tea given in her honor. I'd read that while she'd been in the cave she had practiced yoga daily, so when we met, I shyly asked her about her yoga practice. She just laughed. "Oh, I'm a lazy one! I haven't done yoga once since I left the cave!"

She was scheduled to speak tonight at seven P.M. At six thirty, I was still a couch puddle in sweatpants. David texted me:

D: Where are you?
C: Here.
D: Are you coming?

C: I don't know.

D: You love JTP. I think you should come.

C: . . .

D: I'm already in the meditation hall and I've saved you a cushion. Are you coming?

C: I don't know.

D: Please, please, please come.

C: . . .

I really didn't want to see David or anybody else. But I knew that if I didn't go see Jetsunma, I would regret it, so I dragged my heavy heart off the couch, washed my face, and grabbed a taxi.

I made it to the center just in time to plop down on the meditation cushion David had saved for me and then stand right back up again. Jetsunma was entering the meditation hall. I bowed to show my appreciation and respect as she entered the room.

Of course, she couldn't care less about that and when she got up to the front of the room motioned for everyone to please sit down. Like everyone there, I was riveted by this bald old lady with the wide grin and a look both wrathful and compassionate and definitely full of spit and vinegar.

She began where it always begins in Buddhism, reminding us of the preciousness of human life. "If we could only realize how everything really is changing in every single millisecond . . ." I loved everything she said even if I did space out a little bit. And then her voice cut through my daydreaming.

She said, "Let go. Let go. Let go."

It is said that a sign of a true master meditation teacher is that each person in the audience thinks the teacher is talking just to them. In that moment, I knew she was talking to me. I knew I was holding on to something I really wanted to let go of, but I just didn't know how. I didn't know who I would be without the part of me that judges, that expects perfection. Who would I be if I didn't have my negative story line? Who would I be if I wasn't mad at David and hurt by his betrayal? I couldn't find any kind of clear visualization for that, but I knew that I wanted to find it.

After Jetsunma concluded her talk, I was the second in line to get her book autographed. She had picked up her fountain pen and started writing her name in old-fashioned English calligraphy when her assistant said, "Jetsunma, this is Cyndi Lee, the yoga teacher." She immediately stopped writing and looked up at me with recognition. I was surprised that she remembered me and I felt, as I had before, a genuine connection to her. Her face split into a crooked smile that charmed me, and she squeezed my hand. I was already all cried out or I'm sure I would have started crying again right then. The kindness that came through her soft palm into my hand was something new and I realized I hadn't been the recipient of that kind of genuine caring for much too long, probably since my mom and I had traded places with caretaking.

That night I sent an email to Jetsunma's assistant requesting a private meeting. I knew it was a long shot, and his return email matched my expectation, telling me that the schedule was very tight and it was unlikely since Jetsunma was going out of town and had important meetings with high lamas and rich donors.

Two days later, another email popped up inviting me to meet Jetsunma the next day at four P.M. I confirmed immediately.

It was a 3-H day: hot, humid, and hazy. A committed New York downtowner, I will go to Moscow or Hong Kong or Rome, but I never go above Fourteenth Street unless absolutely necessary. This day I gladly made the pilgrimage up to Forty-Ninth Street to the apartment where Jetsunma was staying. It turned out to be a fancy building, and my arrival was announced by the doorman while I waited for the elevator. I knew you didn't have to dress up for a meeting with a Buddhist nun, but I wanted to show my respect, so along with an armful of flowers, I was wearing a pretty flowered summer dress and gold sandals.

When I stepped off the elevator, Jetsunma was waiting for me, literally with open arms. Her assistant took the flowers so that Jetsunma could put her arms around me as if we were old, dear friends and suddenly we were.

"Would you like some tea? I'm going to have some."

As the assistant nun went to the kitchen to prepare our tea, Jetsunma took my hand and led me over to a love seat where we sat together. She sat sideways on the little sofa in Sukhasana, legs crossed beneath her, so she could face me. It took some negotiating with my slim summer dress but I managed to do the same, and we sat facing each other.

I was a little bit nervous but not terribly because Jetsunma was so friendly she put me at ease. Realized beings are always relaxed. Jetsunma was not out to get anything. She didn't have an agenda. Being around someone that open shifted the atmosphere. There was no need for small talk.

I told her of my suffering, and mentioned feelings of betrayal and rejection, and a lack of clarity about how to move on. I confessed that I wanted to let go but kept getting snagged by my emotions; so much confusion and sadness and anger, too.

"Oh my dear." She took my hands again. She might be a celibate nun, but she knew suffering when she saw it.

"I'm so hurt and lonely and I can't seem to get through to the other side. I'm stuck."

She said the most obvious and perfect thing: "You have to take it into your practice. Turn it into the path." It was encouraging that she thought enough of me as a dharma practitioner to say that. I knew she was right and said so.

"I know you know. That's why you're here." Her advice was gentle but clear. "You have to go to your husband and tell him thank you. 'Thank you for giving me something to work with on my path.'"

I took in a deep breath but didn't respond. I wondered if I could really do that. Wasn't that letting him win? My righteous anger toward him flared up, but Jetsunma wasn't done with the advice.

"And you have to forgive the women, too. You know, they are just lonely women."

I bristled at that, and she saw it, and said, "Oh, this is going to be tough for you."

She rustled around a little bit, reorganized her robes so that she could lean forward and hold my hand again.

"You must practice Maitri for yourself. Loving-kindness. Start to do it every day. You do know how to do that practice?"

"Yes."

"Well, normally you do it for others, but you must do this for yourself right now. Recite these phrases:"

May I be safe,
May I be healthy,
May I be happy,
May I live with ease.

I repeated them with her and then she nodded. "Yes, do this for yourself. This will really help you."

Instantly, I knew she was right. This ancient Buddhist practice of cultivating feelings of loving-kindness was something I'd practiced for many years. It was always popular among my students because it cuts through thinking and goes right to the heart. Whenever I taught it as part of my Yoga Body, Buddha Mind workshops, I would make sure to have plenty of boxes of tissues on hand. Maitri uses the concentration that has been developed from basic mindfulness meditation to focus on positivity toward others. The scripture instructs the practitioner to cultivate specific thoughts of goodwill, compassion, and unconditional friendliness toward all living beings everywhere, without exception. You learn to hold your attention on these thoughts with a soft heart, which the scripture calls a practice of mindfulness and sublime abiding.

The instruction I had originally received was to say the four lines for three living beings: someone you love; someone you are having a problem with; and finally, for someone who is a neutral person to you. It is easy to wish happiness, health, safety, and a life of ease for those you love, but it gets more challenging to do that for someone you don't like, and surprisingly, it is often most difficult for those you feel neutral toward. So the power of this practice is that it wakes us up to the fact that every single living being is like us; we all want to be happy and loved. It's really as simple as that. Once that sensitivity is aroused, we begin to experience our own heart breaking in a beautiful way. This open heart no longer allows us to ignore other people or wish them ill, when we see so clearly that we are all suffering in some way or another already.

One of the concepts around cultivating anything good inside ourselves is that we are a bit like sponges. When we get squeezed or pressured, what we've practiced is what will come out. Just like making imprints in yoga class, these loving-kindness imprints will show up when push comes to shove.

Of course, this takes time and that's why it's called a practice. But *drip, drip, drip,* the bucket fills, and eventually Maitri practice is said to create awakening in the heart of the meditator; and traditionally that is a prerequisite to attaining the state of a bodhisattva.

I'd sent these four lines, like prayers on the wind, to my beloved, difficult, and neutral people many times. I definitely have a sense that practicing Maitri has created loving imprints within me. But it was not the same as coming right out and doing the practice for myself. How had I never thought of that before? A bodhisattva must work for her own liberation, too.

We talked about other things, her need to do more exercise now that she was over sixty, and how wonderful it would be if I could visit her nunnery in India. Maybe I could give the nuns a

yoga teacher training since they already had a daily yoga practice. But the conversation continued to circle back to me and
she stayed consistent in her advice. "Take it onto your path. You
know how to work with obstacle as a path, don't you, my dear?
And don't forget to practice Maitri for yourself."

A generous hour and a half later, we hugged good-bye and
when I hit the street, I didn't care that it was still a 3-H day. I
didn't care that it was five thirty and I was in Midtown, where
getting a taxi is a dog-eat-dog event. I started walking downtown and my gold sandals chewed up my heat-swollen feet, just
as they had in Hong Kong. But I didn't care. It wouldn't last forever, and anyway, the need to find something outside myself as
a landing pad for my hurt seemed to have lifted.

Jetsunma's genuine caring and gentle straightforward manner had been the soft knife that I needed right then to cut
through confusion and open the door to clarity. She not only
helped me untwist my mental Moebius strip, she gave me a new
direction in which to go. Like coming out of a dark movie the-
ater sometimes makes you notice the brightness of the world, I
had a new perspective on my life and another way to live it. It
was about letting go, of course. Letting go of my own habits
that prevent me from feeling safe, happy, healthy, or at ease.

It would take hard work to break the bones of those old
ways of thinking, but I was ready to work with obstacles as my
path. I was ready to pull the plug and let my emotional tsunami
whirlpool down the drain. And I knew I could do it, because
Jetsunma had faith in me and I had faith in her and that equaled
faith in myself.

This inspiration rose up in me as I walked down Second

Avenue, across Twenty-third Street, past my old apartment on Fourteenth Street. As I took a right on Twelfth Street, heading back to my studio, I noticed that I was coated with city schmutz, stuck to my humid skin. But just like the shower that was in my near future, I felt purified inside, too. Finally, my body and my heart felt light.

———— ◆ ————

Maitri gave me a hook to work with. The practice became my new go-to place, instead of where I used to go, which was the "land of negativity and self-judgment." Letting go of thoughts when they arise, even in a friendly "oh, you're here again, but I don't need you anymore" way had really only been the first step.

It was what I had learned in Deer Park and from Rimpoche so many years before. First, we have to recognize our suffering. Then, we acknowledge the cause of suffering, which is always resisting things being as they are. That understanding points the way to the end of suffering, so that you can begin to walk the path of wise and compassionate living. I simply hadn't recognized the road that would lead out of my self-critical perfectionism until Jetsunma pointed it out.

Whether it came to my marriage, my yoga studio, a request for a work commitment, or a meeting with an employee, I started listening even more closely to the sensations in my body. When signals of discomfort arose, such as a bad feeling in my stomach or exhaustion for no good reason, I practiced Maitri. I rarely got past the first two slogans.

"May I be safe" turned out to be much more potent than I'd

thought. When I asked myself what it would take to make me feel safe, my question wasn't about needing physical protection in a dark alley. I felt more endangered in certain relationships, at home and at work. I imagined what it would look like if I felt safe in those situations, and just doing that one thing was such a huge act of kindness to myself that everything began to shift.

It worked the same way with "May I be healthy." I started to recognize the unhealthy habits in my life—overworking, traveling too much, over-committing, and caring too much about what other people might think of me. I admitted to myself that I was afraid of getting overbooked and ending up with an ulcer like I had the year before. I was afraid to return to Tokyo. I had never wanted to admit these kinds of fears before because I thought that buffalo-ing through life meant I was strong and capable. But it was a huge relief to acknowledge what was unhealthy for me—a natural first step toward taking better care of myself in every way. I rejoined the gym, just as I told myself I would, which helped me sleep better, which helped me eat better, which made me feel better about myself.

That old grumpy voice was the one thing not being fed. As she began to dissolve, I had another insight. The most important safe and healthy environment was inside my head. I was no longer willing to live in a place where the law said I had to be perfect. And I was not going to live with someone who didn't like me, respect me, or take proper care of me, so I broke up with that person—the woman who hated her body—and decided to become the kind of person I did want to live with.

Finding happiness and ease seemed to flow naturally from giving myself a guarantee of safety, making the best safe haven my own mind. I felt more relaxed living with a self that loves me—warts and all.

Louise Hay said, "Look in the mirror and say, 'I love you.'" Another favorite teacher of mine, Sakyong Mipham, said, "Look in the bathroom mirror every morning and repeat three times, 'It's not about me.'" Gelek Rimpoche said, "Equanimity begins with you. Treat yourself better. You can't divide yourself into parts and hate one part and love another—both parts are you."

I had come to realize that these words were conveying the same message. I was sick of being sad and mad about being betrayed but I was also sick of thinking about myself so much. I understood that if I took proper care of myself, I would also be taking care of everyone, including my husband and my mom. I needed to cut myself some slack and create my own mental refuge, a place that didn't mind wobbly bits but did mind a life without joy. I saw that I had a path now—one that doesn't just steer me away from the old stuff, but moves me in a compassionate direction. When I had left home at eighteen, my friends said, "You must have really hated your parents," but they'd gotten it all wrong. I loved my parents. I wasn't leaving to get away from them. I was leaving to go toward something, an undertaking full of unknowns, the whole big world. Self-compassion as the foundation for compassion for others was now my new big adventure.

I met David that night and right away he could tell I was happier and more open. He asked me what Jetsunma had said, but I didn't tell him. I couldn't yet get the words out to say thank you for giving me something to work with on my path. But the lightness was still there, lifting my heart.

————— ◆ —————

The Yoga Body, Buddha Mind workshop had come to an end. The core of the OM yoga teachings, this weekend program offers a detailed integration of mindfulness meditation and yoga practice. After learning how to Make Friends with themselves on Friday night, the students practice *Dynamic Equilibrium* and bravely approach Obstacle as Path on Saturday. Following Sunday morning's session called *Awakened Heart*, the teacher training students were once again sitting in a circle with me.

We had gathered in the Space studio, which is the least popular of the five yoga rooms at my center. The design of each studio is based on a natural element: the Earth studio has a terra-cotta-colored ceiling; the blue ceiling in Sky studio expresses the air element; the Sun studio has a saffron ceiling for fire; the Forest studio's avocado-colored ceiling represents the wood element, and the hallways, the areas of traffic flow in between studios, are painted blue for water.

Some people find the Space studio claustrophobic with its low white ceiling and lack of windows, but that's just why I like it. New Yorkers are always desperate for bigger spaces, but of course, it doesn't matter how much external space we inhabit if we don't have space in our minds. So this pristine studio is my little "inner space" statement. It's a meditation cave, offering no distractions to going into deeper aspects of our yoga practice, such as learning how to transmit the practice of yoga through teaching.

The teacher trainees looked different, more processed, than they did at the beginning of their course. Their posture was uplifted, their eyes were clear. They knew exactly how to use their yoga props; everyone was sitting up on at least one meditation cushion or blanket, some people using blocks to support their thighs and relax their hips. As a group they had become more dignified and yet more open.

On this Sunday afternoon, they had me all to themselves. They weren't feeling shy around me anymore. In fact, they were full of questions. What they mostly wanted to ask me were questions we call "What if's?"

Eric started it off. "I have a question about something I saw recently. What if a student totally ignores the teacher and does her own thing in class?"

Everyone laughed, glad he had asked that. They've all seen students act that way and know it can be awkward. They looked to me for the answer.

"Well, there are various things you can do. First of all, you need to make sure that she doesn't have an injury. If she does, of course, you must help her find a safe way to modify her practice."

Maggie nodded. "Yes, absolutely, but what if this person is not injured?"

"Well, instead of singling out that student, you can say something to the whole group. For example, you might mention how wonderful it is to be together that day because one of the main reasons to come to yoga class is to be with other people; to practice wakefulness, compassion, and curiosity in a group setting as a template for how to be in the world. Or"—I got an idea—"how about this? Everybody stand up."

"Us, right now?"

"Yes, everyone stand up and pretend you are not in teacher training right now, but that you are in a regular yoga class."

They stood in Tadasana in front of their cushions: feet together, quadriceps engaged, shoulders balanced directly over hips, gaze steady and alert. They were ready to follow my instructions.

"Inhale and extend your left arm forward straight out in front of you. And exhale, lower your arm down by your side."

These students were so into yoga that even a simple movement like this was intensely interesting to them. They made this gesture with complete attention and precision.

"Now, inhale and extend your right arm straight out in front of you. And"—I took a pause—"walk around and shake hands with three people here who you haven't met before." This got a laugh because, of course, they've been spending every day together for months and months, but the point was made. As they shook one another's hands, Parker said, "I get it! You're building community."

"That's right! And you will all be able to come up with your own creative ways of doing that." Clearly inspired, they sat down on their cushions and began writing in their notebooks.

"Although"—I paused, remembering a challenging situation from years before—"I did have a guy who regularly came to my class and did whatever he wanted. One day he started doing the splits while I was leading a quiet, seated meditation! At the end of that class, I tried to be totally non-aggressive when I asked him why he didn't follow the group instructions. He admitted that he preferred to do his own yoga practice but his apartment was too small, so he had to come to a larger space. It wasn't easy to tell him that he would only be allowed back to class if he was willing to follow the instructions, but it is the teacher's responsibility to hold the space in a way that supports the entire group."

Hands flew up for the next question. "What if a student starts falling in love with you?"

"Well, one thing you can tell them is that lots of people get love feelings when they start practicing yoga, and it's natural to think it's about the teacher. But I think really what's happening is the students are falling in love with themselves."

"Ahhhhh." The teacher trainees nodded and looked at each other in a way that reminded me how much they had all fallen in love with one another during this intense training period. Their training was almost over and they were feeling very tender toward one another. Perhaps that's what brought up the next question.

"What do you do if someone starts crying?"

I knew this question wasn't just theoretical. They had spent that morning learning Maitri practice and the tissues had been plentiful. I turned the question back to them. "What do you think?"

"Give them a tissue."

"Leave them alone."

"Bring them some water."

"Tell them it's okay to cry in yoga, that emotions often come to surface and it's a safe place to feel them."

I let them run through all these options and when they ran out of steam, I gave them a pop quiz: "What is the first thing you look at when making an adjustment in yoga class?"

They went silent for a second, knowing they'd been taught this key point and not wanting to get it wrong. Renate calmly said, "The person."

"Yes. Remember, we're teaching people, not poses."

"Right, right."

"You're almost done with your training. By this point, you've got an excellent bag of tools for working with all kinds of students. But the answer to any of your questions is always going to be the same: 'It depends.' Good teaching is not formulaic. What you do depends on the person in front of you that day and what you feel when you connect with that person. Any of the answers you suggested could be the right one, depending on circumstances. Figuring this out is where your teaching comes alive. Teaching yoga—and living yoga—is not about reproducing anything. It's about seeing what is needed right here, right now."

Heads nodded thoughtfully.

Suddenly, the gap of silence was broken as the Space cave door opened. Cherie, the studio manager, poked her head in. "I'm sorry to interrupt, Cyndi, but it's your mother . . ."

Trying to stay calm and dignified, I excused myself, but once outside the Space studio, I rushed down the blue hallway to take the phone call in my office. My mom's heart rate had dropped to a dangerously low level and the nursing home's interim weekend doctor, who didn't know one thing about my mother, was recommending that she be sent to the emergency room.

"No! Do not take her to the emergency room. I'll be there in twenty minutes."

I knew that doctor was covering herself and I did not want my mother going into the hell realm known as a New York City emergency room.

My own heart was pounding as I zoomed up the highway along the East River, wondering if this was going to be the end. My emotions were tangled and complex. There was a seductive sense of relief that this might be the end of the painful journey for my mom, after which maybe I could get my life back. But I also knew that when my mom passed, I wouldn't get my life back. I'd have a different life, in a world that didn't include my mom. That thought made me deeply sad. When those thoughts collided, I cut them all loose and tucked my legs—still in yoga pants—under me, sitting tall in the backseat. I tried to stabilize my mind by deepening my breathing, which immediately made me realize this taxi had B.O. Just like yoga practice, coming back to sensation when your mind strays wakes you up and returns you to the present. Rolling down the window shocked me out of my cave-mind. My mother might be dissolving, but there were still tugboats on the river, people fishing off the pier, and kids eating street pretzels on this pleasant Sunday afternoon.

The taxi pulled up in front of the nursing home and I jumped out into the sunny day. On either side of the front doors were elderly people swaddled in their wheelchairs, tended by caretakers like Maureen. It was hard to look at them because they seemed so empty of life. Even the well-groomed uptown ladies, who'd been dressed by their daughters in fur-collared coats and cashmere scarves seemed unkempt, which was less about their appearance than the lack of consciousness in their aura. I smiled at them anyway but got no response as I rushed inside the building.

Millie didn't respond to me either. It was unclear whether she was sleeping or in a coma, but the nurse said her condition had already stabilized. Maureen was sitting by the bed, working on her crocheting. She reached over and took Millie's hand. "You should have felt her earlier today. Her skin turned so cold." She started rubbing lotion on those familiar hands. Maureen had already tucked Millie's hair neatly behind her ears and rubbed Vaseline on her lips. Maureen hadn't been able to put a cute T-shirt on her today because she was intubated with IV fluids and oxygen in each nostril.

Maureen looked at me and said, "She's giving up."

It's true that Millie hadn't taken any food for two weeks, but I wished Maureen wouldn't say things like that out loud in front of her.

"Yesterday I saw a woman at the end of the bed. A ghost, dressed in an old-fashioned skirt and blouse. She was pretty." She paused to see whether I thought she was nuts. "Does that sound like it could be your grandmother?"

"I don't know, Maureen. Maybe."

"I think it is. I think your grandmother is visiting Millie. She wants her to come home."

"Maybe, Maureen. I don't know."

David says I have to let my mom go, and I know he's right. But letting go is not the same as giving up, and I'm not ready to give up on her. Neither is Dr. Griffo. He told me she was in renal failure again and may have had a small stroke on Sunday. When the IV fluids and oxygen get her levels up to where she was when she first came to the nursing home, he'll take her off support. Dr. Griffo has persuaded me to let her take the lead at that point. If my mom doesn't accept food and doesn't open her eyes, she will cease to thrive and most likely pass away in a few days. As she is now, she can't walk, she can't speak straight, she can't take solid food, and she can't die. What she can do is dissolve, bit by bit. Her bones are frail, her skin is dry, her breathing is shallow, and her consciousness is leaking away. But Dr. Griffo said her heart is still very strong.

Millie started slipping sideways off her stack of pillows. Maureen got up to adjust her, tucking an extra pillow under her right side, which seemed to even her out. Her hair began to spread out and her nightie slid down one shoulder. If I didn't know her, I'd find her hard to look at, too. I wouldn't think of her as a person who was once vibrant and smart and pretty, a fun mom who taught her five-year-old daughter how to turn cartwheels on the beach. But I do know her and she looks beautiful to me. In fact, the more frail and messy and confused she gets, the more clearly I see her as a person.

I know she wasn't perfect. Like any daughter, I can think of things she could have done better. She could have been more open with me, shared more of her inner life and asked me about mine. She could have been less scared of her own sexuality and less protective of mine. But she was also the cool mom who slipped me the car keys on school nights and thought it was funny when she found condoms in my high school purse, believing me when I told her I had no idea what they were or how they got there.

My mom was all those moms to me, and all of them were here dying in front of me. David said I should tell her she can go, but I don't think she needs me to say that. She has never indicated to me that she wants out, and anyway, she's my mom. I don't tell her what to do; she tells me what to do. She used to talk to me a lot, and often she'd talk to people who weren't actually there. But she's shut down now, and I can't remember the last time she said a word to me. I talked to her anyway and then after sitting with her until dark, I gave her a kiss and went home.

The nursing home was like being in a cave, too. When I exited onto York Avenue, Manhattan pumped life back into me. I walked the streets for a while before catching a cab back home, where I collapsed into bed. I was exhausted, but I couldn't fall asleep. What if Millie died in the night? When I did finally sleep, I had disturbing dreams that made me feel guilty. I woke up feeling wasted, dragged myself out of bed, and made the dreaded trip back uptown.

I slowed down as I entered the nursing home the next morning, nervous about what I would find when I got to Millie's room. Please don't let it be an empty bed! Maureen didn't arrive until eleven A.M. and I didn't really trust the nursing staff to do the right thing, to treat Millie with enough tenderness, to call me if there was a change. I wondered if they were treating patients or people.

But there she was, and nothing had changed. She was alone. Her eyes were closed and she looked peaceful. It was hard to believe she was eighty-six. In a weird way, it's been a gift to be able to care for Millie. As her illness has deepened, so has our relationship. We've become closer, more intimate, more honest with each other. I guess that happens when you have to go into the bathroom stall with your mom to help her with her diapers and make sure she doesn't fall down. And the big fat surprise of it all is that the more I reflect on how my mom raised me, the more faults I see, and the more faults I see, the more I love her. I can only hope she knows that.

I stepped over to the bed. I knew she couldn't respond, but maybe she could still hear me. I whispered, "Hi, Mom." Did I see a slight lift in the corners of her mouth, or did I just imagine a smile? "How about a hug?" I leaned over the hospital bed and scooped my arms under her frail shoulders. When I tenderly placed my face next to hers, it felt as if we were almost the same person. And then, for the first time in many days, she spoke clearly and right out loud: "Love. There's nothing but love." She didn't die that day, but she did speak clearly to me, giving me those words as her final gift.

———— • ✦ • ————

One last sip of coffee and then I had to get a move on. It was time to get ready to teach yoga. I leaned over to fluff up the cushions on the couch, smoothing the wrinkles in the silk and velvet fabric. I had brought the brightly patterned silk all the way home from a roadside fabric shop in India, and it was delicate. It hadn't been easy for me to sew these two slippery fabrics together, and I was really proud of how elegant my cushion creations had turned out. I loved this fabric and didn't want it to get torn. It was worth it to me to take a moment to give proper care to these cushions.

Getting into the shower meant passing the bathroom door, which meant walking past the full-length mirror. I used to say "Ugh!" when I saw my reflection or, on a good day, sigh with disappointment. Today I looked up and smiled at myself. That made me laugh.

Lately I had stopped weighing myself, instead getting feedback about how I felt from, well, how I actually felt. It really wasn't better to look good than to feel good. When I felt good, I almost always looked good, but when I looked good, I didn't necessarily feel good. I had begun to appreciate that life is too short to waste it feeling bad.

I had looked up the numbers. In 2011, an estimated 77 percent of American women and girls thought they were unattractive and had low self-esteem. Other studies showed that this way of thinking leads to destructive behaviors like alcohol and drug use. On any given day in America, 45 percent of women were on a diet; 81 percent of ten-year-old girls were afraid of being fat; 91 percent of college women had tried to control their weight through dieting; and 35 percent of "normal" dieters would become pathological dieters.

Girls with self-esteem issues are having sex younger and younger—not for pleasure but because it makes them feel attractive and loved.

So why was I smiling in the mirror? Because something was

changing with me. When I looked in the glass now, I saw myself and my body—not just *a* body, but *my* body—which is part of me. When I was fourteen, I had hated showing off my new clothes to the church ladies. I still didn't like being appreciated only for my appearance. It created too much pressure and was, I now realized, an incomplete appreciation of a complex female being.

I mourned the objectification of women, propagated by porn and gentlemen's clubs among other social ills, that creates a mind-set in which women are interchangeable and ultimately supports a world where rape and sex trafficking flourish. But if I was going to be totally honest, I had to admit that I also propagated the objectification of women through my own hyperfocus on my body, along with harsh self-judgment, constant comparisons with other women, and jealousy of those younger, thinner, or prettier.

I stepped into the shower and the hot water helped me tune in to my body even more. Every day is different, I realized, and depending on whether I felt light or heavy, loose or tight, tired or refreshed from a good night's sleep, I have an egg for breakfast or cook up some oatmeal. I was getting pretty good at taking proper care of myself, a direct result of liking myself at least as much as the cushions on my couch.

Stepping out of the shower, I thought about my plans for that afternoon. I was going to meet my dear friend Diane at her doctor's office. She had asked me to go with her to her postbreast-cancer-surgery checkup. It was only a few months ago that we were debating whether she should go for chemo or undergo a double mastectomy, a dramatic option, yet one that would reduce the possibility of her developing lymphedema, which could threaten her career as a high-end hair stylist.

We met for dinner, laughing as we hugged and greeted each other with our mutual nickname.

"Hello, my dzolly!"

"Hello, my dzolly!"

She had requested that we eat at Souen, since the menu had many organic, healthy vegetarian options. In a straightforward, non-pushy, non-guilty way, Diane was simply taking proper care of herself through diet, prayer, yoga, and surrounding herself with loved ones. I was happy to support her by eating at Souen and wondered why I couldn't do as good a job expressing my needs without feeling selfish.

I always learned a lot from Diane and that's one of the reasons we had been friends since the late, great eighties in the East Village. She had done my hair for my first wedding—a short, black, spiky do with a tiara. Another time she dyed my two-inch hair blond with a long, fluffy turquoise fringe in the front. A few marriages, many apartments, and even more gigs later, we still looked to each other for help in making important decisions. We were the executors in each other's wills, and we were always there for each other, no matter what, no questions asked, no judgments made.

"Can I start you off with a drink?" The waitress interrupted at just the right moment. After reviewing her upcoming surgery options, Diane had just asked me what was new in my world. I hadn't told any of my friends about the book I was writing, although Mary came close to guessing. I had learned that talking too much about a new project could disperse my focus and energy. But I wanted to tell Diane about it because I trusted her to keep a secret. I also thought she would be a great person with whom to discuss body hatred and confused self-perception. Over the years she had experimented with a wide repertoire of clothing styles, including dressing like a man in public. Tonight she looked lovely and slim in a pair of jeans and a pretty spring blouse.

I had been just about to tell her about my I Hate My Body book project when the waitress interrupted. That momentary gap in our conversation was just long enough for my intuition and compassion to kick in. I realized that there was no way I could tell this woman who was battling breast cancer how much energy I had been expending over the years complaining about my looks and my legs and all those other parts of me that were actually perfectly fine and perfectly healthy. What was I thinking?

As Diane calmly ordered Mu tea, I held back tears. "Mu tea for me, too, please," I said. The waitress left and I told Diane about some exciting yoga gigs I had coming up. She didn't know it, but Diane had just taught me something new. Through all the years of dancing, working out, practicing yoga, I had never really cut through the ambition to make my body look better, never let go of dissatisfaction with my appearance. But looking at her open face, full of goodness during a time of such tough choices, I realized how fortunate I actually was.

There is a famous Buddhist story about a man who has lost his fortune. He looks everywhere for it, never realizing it has been under his floorboards all along. The message is that we already have what we need, but we are stuck in the cycle of suffering, a pervasive feeling of dis-ease that we think is solid and can't let go of.

But there is a hidden treasure in all of us all the time. Our spiritual practices—yoga, mindfulness meditation, Maitri practice—offer us paths for uncovering the treasure within, our own Basic Goodness. The sticky stuff inside us that we thought was just a clod of dirt begins to shine and turns out to be a nugget of gold. Sweep the dust and sweep the dirt.

———— ✦ ————

Seiko is filled with craving for a handstand. A regular in my Tuesday intermediate class where we work on inversions, she wants to do a handstand so bad that when I say, "Okay, everybody take your mats to the wall for handstands," I can see her mind and body turn into a fist. Her focus is not the useful kind, but more like an obsession.

I work with her every week, trying to get her to slow down, to incorporate mindfulness into her efforts, to be interested in her process. I know this is what she needs in order to understand herself—where she is clear and where she is confused, where her leg is in space and why that is not going to take her upside down the way she wants.

"Stay steady for a moment, Seiko, and just feel what it's like to be you right now in this shape." She sighs loudly, not unlike my dog when I tell him to sit and stay.

I share a personal story in an effort to inspire Seiko and the whole class: "My dad taught me to drive at the shopping mall. This was back in the day when malls used to close at 7 P.M. After dinner we would go to the mall parking lot, which was empty and therefore, the perfect place for me to learn to drive our German car with the heavy stick shift and clunky pedals. Again and again, I stalled the car and then jerked it forward, grinding the gears as my dad grinded his teeth. But eventually I got the hang of it. Soon he allowed me to drive on the quiet side streets. And now? I'm all grown up and I can drive all by myself on the interstate highways! Get it? Yes, it's because I went slowly at first that I was later able to keep my awareness at eighty miles per hour."

I try to get my students to understand that we are going slowly through the preparation for each pose so that we can find out when and where we go off track. Later, when your mind and body are more clearly aligned you can just kick right up. But for now, what they are practicing is paying attention to their habits, to noticing when they occur, and in that very moment, to making choices about how they want to relate to those patterns.

I think this goes in one of Seiko's ears and out the other. She jumps up and down and up and down, getting frustrated. I could talk about how we all create our own suffering but perhaps that would not be well received right now. Teachers need to pick their spots, too.

But I wonder how I can help Seiko to slow down enough to feel what she is doing. If she did, she would be surprised to realize that she is already doing a handstand. She's already got what she wants. It's just that she kicks up so hard that she ends up banging her foot into the wall every time, which rebounds her off the wall and right back down to the floor. It all happens so fast she doesn't even know she's up before she is back down. She thinks she needs to work harder, do more, even though I tell her to take it easier, to do less. I know that is the only way she will feel the connections. But for now, she is stuck on the end point, which is why she was super-excited when she finally made it all the way up into a handstand the other day. "Cyndi, I'm up! I'm up!" she squealed in class and then promptly fell down again.

I'm the teacher; my job is to be helpful. What Seiko needs now is a boost up, just like Louise offered to me. I walk over to the wall ready to catch her legs the next time she kicks up. I'll hold her up in her balance long enough for her to feel that she already has what she has been wanting so badly. If she can get a flash of awareness, a mini-satori, it will plant a seed that might help her suffering dissolve, at least for a few breaths.

⁕

The ficus plant in my corner window has managed to keep itself alive for decades. It lives by the window in the house that once belonged to David's mother, out on the east end of Long Island. Nowadays it's our private retreat spot; we call it our happy place. We New Yorkers get used to living in a pressure cooker where we are in constant negotiation with buses, bikes, umbrellas, and way too many people just to get across the street. The prevalent nature experience of the city is human nature and, of course, doggy nature. Out here there is open space and more than just a patch of sky. The minute we arrive, I feel my skin expand and my brain fist relax.

I opened the door to the backyard for Leroy to go out, then started in on my comforting arrival rituals, which included taking care of The Plant. Since it's the only one we have, I'd feel bad if it croaked from lack of attention. That's why it's a good plant for me. Sometimes weeks pass between our visits here, but all I have to do is slowly empty a full pitcher of water on The Plant whenever I return, and it starts to thrive again.

I walked over to the kitchen where the red-and-yellow-striped vintage pitcher that David and I had bought together at a flea market was sitting on the windowsill. As I filled it with water, I thought back to my experience in the big earthquake. I'd been home long enough to process some of it, and I felt grateful that nothing much had happened to me except for some inconvenience and a bit of upset. I'd been worried about my friends in Japan but they had written that they were okay and things were pretty much returning to normal.

David went outside to walk around the yard, checking to make sure the fence was still intact and Leroy couldn't get out. The sun was just starting to set between the still-bare branches. I felt sadness rise, I touched the feeling of that, and then I watched it start to dissolve.

I walked over to the corner window, tucked the lip of the pitcher into the thicket of ropy strands around the ficus's mini-trunk, and let it start drinking. The ficus didn't seem mad that I hadn't been there sooner. It didn't seem to have abandonment issues or to hold a grudge. It accepted the water. As I moved the pitcher to the other side of the big clay pot and poured, I saw fresh green buds peeking out. Empty pitcher on the floor, I knelt down and gently tugged off the dried-up leaves and stalks so the babies could get the nourishment they needed.

That's one thing I had learned from the earthquake, the tsunami, and the unsuccessful attempts to stop the nuclear power plant fires: fighting a situation is not as effective as meeting it. Our first impulse might be to fight, to hit back, to meet aggression with aggression. But the earth and all the other elements—water, fire, air, and space—they aren't aggressive. They aren't trying to hurt us. They are just doing what they do. Finding the courage to stay steady and meet the situation as it is, without running away or running toward—this was the message I tried to bring home.

Just as I was walking back to the kitchen, David stepped inside, waited a moment for little Leroy to follow him in, and slid the door shut. He followed me in and we put our arms around each other, another one of our arrival rituals that naturally occurs because we are so happy and grateful to be here in this restful, beautiful place.

Almost right away, I stiffened because I remembered that I was mad at David. I was working through my feelings and I'd come to understand that I didn't always feel safe hugging him. Touching the front of your body to the front of another person's body, even your own husband's, is a vulnerable thing to do and that can be scary. I whispered to myself, "May I be safe, May I be healthy, May I be happy, May I live with ease." That relaxed me.

I still didn't know what was going to happen in my life, but then again, do we ever know, really? No one knew that earthquake was going to happen, or all the other known and unknown results of that event, which are still unfolding and will continue to unfold for years and years. It's a big vinyasa; everything that happens plants a seed and everything that is happening is the fruit of a previous seed. I'm becoming more aware of the seeds I'm planting, and I'm becoming more aware of the seeds that have created my current experiences. That also means I can choose which seeds I want to water. Interdependence includes everything, so everything always matters; every thought, word, and action on the spectrum of arising, abiding, and dissolving. Without dissolving, I reminded myself, we can't grow again.

My Maitri practice has been growing a new highway inside my mind/heart and I have pretty much forgiven myself for being so mean to me. That habit is dissolving. And I have stayed in the hug. Louise Hay's voice comes back to me: "When you get it, you're going to get it for everyone."

Maybe everyone included David, too. If I can forgive myself, maybe I can forgive him. Being in his arms felt like being in another kind of home, another kind of happy place. With my arms encircling his big body, I felt like a human prayer wheel as I whispered to him, "May you be safe, May you be healthy, May you be happy, May you live with ease."

———— ✦ ————

The reason I can teach so many classes is that I keep up my own yoga practice. After all, you can't clean the floor with a dirty mop. Nearly every day you can find me down on my hands and knees, or upside down on my head, stretching and strengthening on that special piece of rubber that some call a yoga mat and I call my magic carpet.

Each time is different but the beginning is always the same. Inhale. Then I exhale and begin my practice, perhaps starting with a balancing breath exercise or a body awareness scan.

But today I reached over and pushed play. After teaching so much lately, I needed a break. I was happy to let someone else teach and to be a student following her lead. The DVD started up, and there I was teaching an OM yoga class.

This DVD had been filmed eight years earlier, and before I caught it, I thought, "Ahk! I've gotten so much older! I was so firm and smooth and fit back then." Non-aggressively but firmly, I escorted that thought out of my head and began to take my own yoga class with the body I had right now.

As instructed by my video self, I drew attention to the physical sensations that always arise, abide, and transform as I moved through simple seated stretches into a series of Sun Salutations. I was comforted by the natural feeling of honest heat that grew gradually with continuous motion. The radiant warmth softened up the stiffness of the old dance injuries that lingered in my right wrist and left knee. The tightness in my neck reminded me of the whiplash I got from a sexy dance video move, but I breathed into it, and that hard spot began to melt, too.

Another memory came up. I remembered that while making this yoga DVD, I threw a drama queen fit about having to wear the microphone on the waistband of my yoga pants. For at least six weeks prior to the shoot, I had cut out all sugar, alcohol, bread, grains, and dairy so that I would look as good as I did that day. And then the director told me I had to wear a wide, fat belt holding a heavy metal box, all of which made my waist look thick. The weight of the box pulled down the front of my pants and I thought it made me look like I had a potbelly. And, as usual, I was not happy with the shape and size of my body, anyway. I took care to hide my butt by walking backward or sideways as I moved among the video yoga students. I stood sideways to disguise my schwahangas.

But now, eight years later, I could see that the microphone did not make my waist look thick at all. In fact, I looked terrific. The habitual moment of being jealous of my own ex-body quickly turned into compassion for that person, that me who was so unhappy about all the wrong things.

Could I apply that compassion to myself right now? The first burn of muscular effort in my legs showed up during the fierce standing pose sequence. This sensation was so well-known to me that I was able to relax into it, as if we were old friends. My body and I have always been a team, and we have done this dance together for decades. Thankfully, struggle was no longer part of my yoga practice.

Momentarily, I spaced out, which made me lose my balance. As I began to topple out of Tree Pose, my DVD self said, "We don't care if we fall over, right? Trees fall over all the time." Hey, how did she know that was exactly what I needed to hear?

This DVD yoga teacher is pretty good, I thought—perceptive, clear, and compassionate. I was actually still using some of this material in my classes but I also knew that I was a much better teacher now. I had the confidence of eight additional years of experience under my belt.

Another thing I had gained in those years was the commitment to stop criticizing myself. If I thought I looked bad then, when obviously I looked good, I was not going to tell myself I looked bad now so that I could regret that eight years into the future.

These arms that could hold my whole body upside down for five minutes—I was not going to call them flabby.

And these legs that could hold a fierce Warrior Pose—why call them squishy? And what about my stomach in Boat Pose? It was the same V-sit shape we used to call the John F. Kennedy President's Fitness Club, and I knew I still could do that core builder until the cows came home.

It was time for backbends, and I decided to ignore my own instructions. Instead of doing three beginner backbends, I went for ten advanced versions. Backbending is often called heart opening, so I decided to combine it with Maitri practice. Each time I pressed my chest to the sky, turning my body into an inside-out version of Brunelleschi's Duomo, I said someone's name out loud.

The first time I said my own name, "Cyndi." In between backbends, I rested on my back and whispered:

"May you be safe
May you be happy
May you be healthy
May you live with ease."

On an inhale I went back up and exhaled the name of my precious teacher: "Gelek Rimpoche."

The third time up was for someone I loved unconditionally. That was easy. "Millie." Exhale and I was back down.

Resting for five breaths, I placed my hands on the front of my body and felt my blood pulsing in my belly and my chest. It felt like my whole body was my heart.

Up I went again, and as I exhaled, I tried to think of the name of a difficult person, but here I got stuck. At that moment, I was not feeling negative and I wondered if my theory was really right, that you can't feel hatred, jealousy, or anger when your chest is this open and vulnerable. I exhaled and came down.

The backbend I was doing, commonly called Wheel, is a big, full-bodied pose. It takes most people a couple of years to accomplish because it requires coordination, strength, and flexibility in your spine, hips, and shoulders. I had that all going on right now. My body, breath, and mind were in a rhythm, and my skin and muscles and bones were working in alignment. Each Wheel gets easier, looser, and stronger at the same time.

254 ✦ Cyndi Lee

I devoted the last six backbends to neutral people. I did not know their names but I could think of plenty of people I had passed by during my day. As the backbends kept unfolding, it occurred to me that there were an immeasurable number of beings to whom I wanted to send wishes of safety, health, happiness, and ease. But ten backbends was enough for today, and anyway, I remembered what Louise Hay had told me: "You can't do everyone."

I met back up with the DVD yoga class, moving through twists, forward bends, and a shoulder stand. Then my yoga teacher told me to lie down on my back for a period of relaxation. I slid the hair elastic off my ponytail, and my shiny, thick, gray hair fanned out around my shoulders.

This is called Savasana, Corpse Pose, traditionally one of the most important asanas of yoga practice. My teacher voice told me that Savasana allows the physical body to cool down and thoroughly digest the benefits of practice. In this position, the earthly body absorbs the seeds planted in the previous poses and starts to bear fruit.

At a more profound level, Corpse Pose gives us the opportunity to practice for the moment what we will all face, the experience of becoming a corpse. When we practice Corpse Pose, we acknowledge that we are only temporarily renting this body, and that some day we will have to let it go. Ironically, Savasana is about embodying the experience of no longer having a body.

Lying in this pose was a good time to reflect on the seeds I had planted. Ending my practice session with Savasana helped me embrace more fully the understanding that I am meant to age and change. How fortunate I am to have experienced so much in these bones. As my body relaxed into the floor, my mind relaxed into the acceptance that my life, like every life, is a flowing vinyasa that arises, abides, and, ultimately, dissolves.

I haven't come into the pose completely yet. I'm lying on my back. My legs have fallen open in a natural way, and I've started to do the "work" of this pose, which is letting go of all physical effort. The instructions for Savasana also include letting go of mental focus. So I let my mind wander and observe my thoughts with a light touch, as if I were watching birds playing in the sky. But I was taking my time putting my arms into the traditional alignment alongside my body.

Of their own accord, my hands came to rest on my upper chest and my attention followed. I liked the way my hands felt on my chest. It was comforting to feel the constancy of my own breath and the rising and falling of my hands as they rode the tides of the air ocean.

And I liked the way my chest felt under my hands. The muscles were firm and my skin was soft. As I moved my hands around that area, a familiar sensation began to arise. I touched my collarbone, a place that had always felt elegant, and that sense of familiarity grew stronger. It was because I had been here before so many times. This lovely place of strength and vulnerability, the moist feeling of my après-yoga skin, the quieting of my breathing pattern—this felt like home.

Of course it did. This was the body I use to work, to play, and to rest. This body was the vehicle, the only vehicle that could take me along my spiritual path. I could not get enlightened—or kinder, more compassionate, more stable, truly happy—until I stopped trying to get rid of the body that I had.

I realized that I had decided to accept the assignment of working with this body. Not to get rid of it; not to resent it; not to wish I looked more like somebody else; but to take this body as it was at this moment on the path toward more goodness.

I knew it didn't have to be perfect, but right then, it felt perfect and I was content. All the bodies I've ever had were here with me right now.

The young body, the too-skinny body, the aerobics-teacher body, the lying-in-bed-after-sex body, the aging body, the partied-too-much body, the sore-muscles body—they were all with me all the time.

I lay quietly and calmly, letting yoga heal me, as it always did, because it's not about thinking but always about feeling. And what did I feel? I felt love. I loved my body. Maybe I would not feel this way all the time, but right then, I did.

I didn't want to be different because I knew there was nothing wrong with me. I knew this because my bones and blood and breath were telling me through the skin of my hand, which felt the beating of my heart. I felt right and good in my body—this body that I had been given for this lifetime and thank you very much. It had done a good job for me so far. Since this was the only container within which I could experience happiness, I wanted to take good care of it, no matter what size or shape it was. If I loved it unconditionally, I might learn to love myself unconditionally, and then to spread this unconditional love to others. That was a good day's yoga practice.

An OM yoga Class for You

Siggy had been taking private yoga lessons from me for a couple of years, but when she came to my apartment on this day she had a problem. The issue was that she wanted to do yoga more often—specifically, on the weekends when she was at her country house. The previous weekend her husband had told her that she was being very crabby and he begged her to go into the other room and do some yoga. Even though he did not practice yoga himself, he had noticed that yoga made Siggy nicer to live with and she knew he was right. So she went into the other room, bent in half, took a few breaths in and out, then lifted her leg and put her foot up on the windowsill. Then she stood there and said to herself, "Now what the heck should I do?"

That was all the motivation I needed to start drawing yoga sequences for students to practice on their own. The only problem was that I didn't really know how to draw. So I did my best, coming up with simple stick figures that worked well enough to communicate the shape and energy of each pose.

After these stick figures were turned into a couple of books—OM yoga: A Guide to Daily Practice and OM yoga Today—people often asked me if I made the stick figures because I wanted to show people that anyone can do yoga. That's not why I started doing them but it's one of the reasons I continued drawing yoga stick figures.

It's pretty easy to feel intimidated by photos of goddess-like yoginis with one leg over their shoulder, doing postures that seem out of reach and out of the question for a normal person with an average body and modest yogic aspirations. These stick figures are meant to cut through any tendency to compare yourself to another person, especially if that person is a professional yoga expert/model.

So, here is a gift to you from me: A basic yoga practice that can be done by almost anyone of any size and shape and experience, including absolute yoga virgins. I hope it will help you connect to your body in a friendly way that is not about how you look but always about how you feel.

———— •◆• ————

Directions for the OM yoga
Warm-Up Sequence:

Take a comfortable cross-legged seat on a small cushion or folded blanket.

Inhale slowly for 4 counts.

Exhale slowly for 4 counts

Repeat this 3 times, always breathing in and out through your nose.

Begin the warm-up sequence by inhaling and alternate exhaling with each position.

1. Inhale, interlace your fingers and reach your palms up to the ceiling.

2. Exhale, bend your elbows, place your hands behind your head and look up, opening your chest.

3. Inhale, reach your palms back up to the ceiling.

4. Exhale, round your back as you press your palms forward, away from your chest.

5. Inhale, arms up next to your ears, fingers reaching to the ceiling.

6. Exhale, twist to the right.

7. Inhale, arms up to the ceiling.

8. Exhale, twist to the left.

9. Inhale, interlace your fingers behind you and lift your chest up to the sky.

10. Exhale, release your arms forward as you fold over your legs.

11. Inhale, round up through your spine, lean back, and balance on your sitting bones with your fingertips on the floor behind you (the seed of the John F. Kennedy Fitness Club pose!).

12. Exhale, sit tall with your hands in prayer in front of your chest.

Repeat three times.

OM YOGA WARM-UP

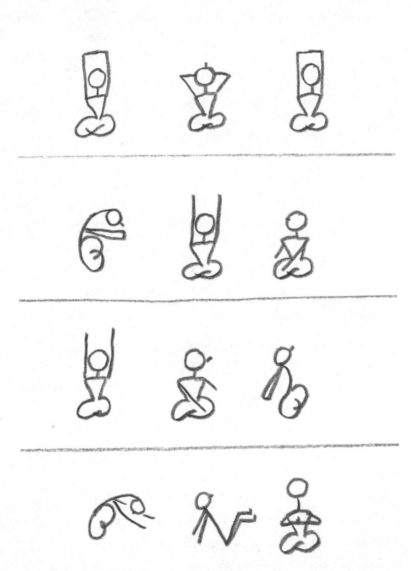

Acknowledgments

————◆————

This book has morphed from a breakfast conversation into a dharma book into a memoir, which means that a lot of people listened to me talk about this thing for a long time.

Thanks must first go to Amy Hertz, my dharma sister and editor of *Yoga Body, Buddha Mind*, for recognizing my essay "I Hate My Body" as the seed syllable for a book that I should write.

A warrior's bow to my friend and agent, Stephanie Tade, who has ridden the stormy waves of samsara with me and helped me get to the other shore with this project.

Much appreciation, gratitude, and respect to my editor, Denise Roy, not just for nudging me to write more and keeping me on track, but for being able to do an awesome handstand in the middle of the room.

An anjali bow to dear Brenda Rosen, who shepherded this project to deadline by fine-tuning my work and even more by being an inspiring dharma teacher and a loving friend.

My knitting pal and author Adrienne Martini actually volunteered to read my book in progress. I bravely emailed her an early, incomplete draft, which she printed out and sent back to me with markings, because she is also a writing teacher. Those notes woke me up and enriched my writing a lot. Thanks and woot.

Namo Jetsunma Tenzin Palmo, for reminding me that obstacles are not a problem; they are always part of the path; in fact, they are the path.

Thank you to Dr. Christiane Northrup. You made me laugh so much, and you were right about everything. The time for flowing shakti is here!

Thank you to my friend Jamie Lee Curtis, for being your smart, big-hearted, and totally honest self and for reminding us to stop worrying about things that don't matter.

Thank you to Louise Hay, for making it personal in the fiercest and most friendly way.

I know the best way for me to thank my dear guru, Gelek Rimpoche, for all that he has given me and continues to give me, is to keep my commitments and do my daily practice. I promise to be a better disciple, Rimpoche.

Thank you to my earthquake friends, especially Brad Bateman, for your natural strength, stability, and clarity.

Namaste and thanks to the thousands of yoga students all over the world who have willingly opened to the OM yoga practice of vinyasa, precise alignment, and Buddhist meditation methods of mindfulness and compassion. You are my dots of awareness and my seeds of inspiration.

David gets more than a thank-you, more than an acknowledgment, more than a low bow to the floor, for continuing to meet me just like always and never the same.

May all beings have happiness and the causes of happiness.
May all beings be free from suffering and the causes of suffering.
May all beings never be parted from freedom's true joy.
May all beings dwell in equanimity, free from attachment and aversion.